SURGICAL PRACTICE ILLUSTRATED

David B. Skinner, Series Editor

ATLAS OF LIVER SURGERY

Christoph E. Broelsch, M.D.

Professor and Chairman
Department of Surgery
University of Hamburg
University Hospital Eppendorf
Hamburg, Germany

Illustrated by Todd Buck

CHURCHILL LIVINGSTONE
New York, Edinburgh, London, Madrid, Melbourne, Tokyo

Library of Congress Cataloging-in-Publication Data

Broelsch, Christoph E.
    Atlas of liver surgery / Christoph E. Broelsch ; illustrated by
Todd Buck.
        p. cm.—(Surgical practice illustrated)
    Includes index.
    ISBN 0-443-08733-4
    1. Liver—Surgery—Atlases.   I. Title. II. Series.
    [DNLM: 1. Liver—surgery—atlases. WI 17 B865a 1993]
    RD546.B76 1993
    617.5′56—dc20
    DNLM/DLC
    for Library of Congress   93-3588
                                        CIP

© Churchill Livingstone Inc. 1993

Distributed in the United Kingdom by Churchill Livingstone, Robert Stevenson
House, 1–3 Baxter's Place, Leith Walk, Edinburgh EH1 3AF, and by associated
companies, branches, and representatives throughout the world.

Accurate indications, adverse reactions, and dosage schedules for drugs are provided
in this book, but it is possible that they may change. The reader is urged to review the
package information data of the manufacturers of the medications mentioned.

Acquisitions Editor: *Robert A. Hurley*
Copy Editor: *Lorene K. Johnson*
Production Supervisor: *Sharon Tuder*
Cover Design: *Gloria Brown*

Printed in the United States of America

First published in 1993   7 6 5 4 3 2 1

Introduction to the Series

Although I originally turned down the prospective North American editorship of an international surgical multispecialty atlas series several years ago, I subsequently thought a lot about the merits of surgical atlases. Given the right circumstances to create an optimal series, the concept is very attractive. The conditions that create the setting and need include the recognition of the rapidly changing nature of surgery, the impact of these changes on formal surgical education, and technical developments to advance the quality of such atlases. When Churchill Livingstone proposed that the time was right for a new atlas series, I agreed with enthusiasm.

Changes in the practice and techniques of surgery in the last 25 years have been phenomenal. Inspecting operating lists for several days in major surgical centers quickly establishes that about 90 percent of the operations done in 1988 were either unknown or could not be done safely when I was in mid-residency in 1963. The rapid introduction of so much new knowledge has inevitably led to fragmentation and specialization. In 1963 at the Massachusetts General Hospital, the general surgery chief residency included independent operating experience in cardiac, colorectal, gynecologic, pediatric, plastic, thoracic, and vascular surgery. Today, each has its own formal specialty certification and residency review process. Included within regular general surgery training were endocrine, fracture, gastrointestinal, hand, hepatobiliary, intensive care, oncology, pancreatic, transplantation, and trauma surgery. Each of these is now offered as specialty fellowships in some hospitals and is evolving toward formal specialty recognition. Neurosurgery, orthopaedics, otolaryngology, and urology were already separate residency programs, but rotation at the junior level exposed the general surgery resident to the principles of each. The breadth of exposure to the techniques and precepts evolving in multiple specialties equipped the resident of that era with a versatility that could be applied to the more rapid evolution of the subspecialty in which he (women were almost nonexistent in surgical residencies 25 years ago) was interested. However, today, no surgeon trained in that era practices the full range of surgery that he learned in residency.

Specialization has become inevitable, and the strong forces driving it continue. The rapid growth in fundamental biomedical knowledge and its application to clinical medicine make it impossible to keep up with new advances in several disciplines. Public interest and knowledge about advances in medicine and surgery have led to a common expectation of specialized expertise. This trend has been reinforced by the credentialing procedure of leading hospitals and the risk of malpractice litigation when difficult problems are taken on by the nonspecialist no matter how able. The rapid emergence in specialization in internal medicine and nonsurgical disciplines led to referral patterns rewarding to the counterpart surgical specialist. Medical school appointments and promotions depend largely on scientific and scholarly contributions that almost by definition require focus and specialization. Finally, modern transportation is such that it is unlikely that a patient with an unusual or complicated problem is more than two hours away from a knowledgeable specialist in that problem.

On the other hand there continue to be factors encouraging more general knowledge and practice in surgery. Specialization carried to extremes is very costly to society. The total cost of medical care in the United States has reached the point where powerful forces are demanding restraint and reversal. This movement places more value on the surgeon who has breadth in his or her armamentarium. For example, HMOs, introduced as a vehicle to contain medical costs, cannot afford to employ full-time specialists in every surgical discipline, yet they have strong economic disincentives to refer out surgery on a fee for service basis. The result is that a true generalist in surgery is highly desirable and busy in an HMO practice setting. Also many procedures which were initially difficult have now become routine, safe, and readily practiced by a generalist.

As operations in the newer disciplines become standardized, they can be done as well and safely in a local setting as in the referral center. A significant portion of the public will choose the local hospital and is encouraged to do so by the local physician who will remain involved in the case. Yet, as pointed out above, these smaller population bases cannot support the full range of subspecialists; therefore, surgeons practicing in the community hospitals should remain up-to-date in several fields and add that which is becoming standardized and routine in related specialties to their own scope of practice.

The explosion in medical and surgical knowledge has extended the benefits of surgical correction to many disorders that are not life-threatening, but that interfere with function and enjoyment of life. When life or limb are at stake, higher risks are acceptable, and the surgical procedure is done with available resources and talents. However, an operation for reconstructive surgery or prophylaxis against future illness must have minimal risks, and the functional success of the operation must be carefully evaluated. This places renewed emphasis on the details of technical surgery and assessment of its impact on the operative results. In recent times, new information on the body's responses to trauma and stress has encouraged emphasis in residency programs in intensive care practice, resuscitation, and the understanding of biochemistry, pharmacology, immunology, nutrition, and sepsis. Yet, at the same time, the evolution of surgical specialties is based substantially on technical innovations and understanding of the effect of these on tissue healing and function.

What has all this to do with the assertion that the setting and time are right for a new surgical atlas series? A medical textbook, and especially a surgical atlas, is essentially an educational tool. The assertion of need must be based on educational grounds. All of the above described changes occurring in surgery have impacted directly on both residency and continuing surgical education. The rapid and recent growth in surgical knowledge and technique means that most active surgical practitioners do not have personal experience and instruction in a number of newer valuable techniques that are being well established. The inevitable conservatism and tradition of residency programs and faculty often means that new techniques developed and taught elsewhere are not rapidly and uniformly evaluated and introduced into a particular program. The numbers of specialties evolving makes it unlikely that any one medical center and surgical residency can afford, or indeed has, up-to-date leadership in each discipline.

The value of cross-fertilization of ideas and techniques across disciplines is well appreciated, but difficult to achieve as barriers are erected among the specialties. With much emphasis appropriately placed in surgical residencies on the scientific basis and acquisition of knowledge in treating shock, infection, and immunologic and nutritional disorders, there is an understandable tendency in some programs to divert attention from or downplay the importance of technique. Yet much of the critical outcome of the newer surgery for non-life-threatening conditions depends directly on surgical technique. An optimally presented multispecialty surgical atlas series can help to address each of these concerns in the surgical residency experience and to support the surgeon desiring to acquire surgical knowledge and techniques in his practice after completion of residency.

Ideally, a surgical atlas series should offer a general education in surgery. Each component of the series should be taught by a world authority in that specialty who has personal experience and judgment to know the variety of techniques available and to select the one most appropriate for the condition at hand and most likely to give the best technical result. In this series, the authors of each volume are surgeons personally known to me as well as generally acknowledged to be technical masters and world authorities in their specialty. Each has significant, scientific contributions to the establishment and advancement of the specialty. Each has published extensively—describing the indications, rationale, and long-term follow-up results of the techniques illustrated. The reader can easily confirm the applicability and validity of the operations described in the published literature and have confidence in its value in his or her practice. As a result, the text of the atlas can be brief, highly technical, and of the utmost practical value to the surgical resident or practitioner who seriously wishes to add excellent techniques to his or her practice base.

In parallel with the developments in surgery, surgical illustration has developed considerably in recent years and is now a more precise discipline. Although artistically gifted surgeons have illustrated their publications for centuries, formal surgical illustration is a more recent event. Max Brodel is generally acclaimed as the founder of the field of medical illustration and established the first school at Johns Hopkins University School of Medicine in 1913. Several other schools became prominent between the first and second world wars. The field acquired greater breadth, sophistication, and rapid growth after the second world war. Today artists are available to do a surgical atlas series soundly based upon detailed anatomic knowledge and personal observation of techniques in the operating room. For this series, a few such highly qualified surgical illustrators have been selected so that a high standard, based both upon artistic excellence and detailed anatomic and surgical knowledge, can be maintained throughout the series.

The changing nature of surgical practices and education, the willingness of world class operating surgeons to participate, the availability of excellent scientifically grounded surgical illustrators, plus the willingness of the publishers to provide a budget to support a top quality surgical atlas series have proved irresistible to me. I hope the product will prove immensely useful to many colleagues in all surgical disciplines who stand to learn and benefit greatly from the techniques that world authorities in related surgical fields have to offer.

David B. Skinner, M.D.
President and Chief Executive Officer
Attending Surgeon
The New York Hospital
Professor, Department of Surgery
Cornell University Medical College
New York, New York

Foreword

Surgical Practice Illustrated is proud to present this seventh volume in the series, the *Atlas of Liver Surgery* by Christoph E. Broelsch. It is a distinguished addition to the series that includes the *Atlas of Vascular Surgery* by Christopher K. Zarins and Bruce L. Gewertz, the *Atlas of Congenital Cardiac Surgery* by Paul A. Ebert, the *Atlas of Adult Cardiac Surgery* by William A. Gay, Jr., the *Atlas of Esophageal Surgery* by David B. Skinner, the *Atlas of Gastric Surgery* by Michael J. Zinner, and the *Atlas of Biliary Surgery* by John L. Cameron. This series emphasizes the selection of an author who is master surgeon with great experience and whose technical approach can be illustrated by an experienced medical artist.

In the past decade, advances in liver surgery have been remarkable. Previously viewed as a difficult and frequently inoperable diseased organ, the recent successes achieved in liver transplantation have made the treatment of serious liver disease a reality. The familiarity with the right upper quadrant achieved through sophisticated biliary and liver surgery has led to new surgical procedures in which the liver can be operated on by its segments, a technique that was developed for lung surgery 50 years ago. A full range of the newly established technical features for segmental liver resection are thoroughly demonstrated in this Atlas.

Professor Christoph Broelsch of the University of Hamburg is a pioneer in these advances in liver surgery and ideally suited to present this Atlas. During his education and training at the University of Hanover in Germany, Professor Broelsch decided to concentrate on liver disease and its treatment by liver transplantation. Fifteen years ago he emerged as one of the most highly regarded and experienced liver transplantation surgeons in Europe. His research focused on the surgical anatomy of the liver and liver preservation. It also led to the scientific background for related donor segmental liver transplantation. Dr. Broelsch was among the first in the world to perform successfully related donor segmental liver transplantation while serving at the University of Chicago.

When I was the Chairman of the Department of Surgery at the University of Chicago, it was my good fortune to be able to recruit Dr. Broelsch from Hanover to Chicago where he established a premier liver transplantation program. The program attracted patients with severe liver disease, many of whom proved to have problems that were amenable to liver surgery without transplantation. Accordingly, Dr. Broelsch's experience with all types of liver surgery increased rapidly, and he has made important contributions to technical liver surgery in addition to his monumental contributions to liver transplantation. Not only is Dr. Broelsch a superb liver surgeon and scientific innovator in this field, but he has also proved to be a master teacher as well. A number of his fellows and residents now hold important positions in major medical schools in North America and Europe and are further advancing the knowledge and treatment of the diseases in the right upper quadrant of the abdomen.

Several years ago, Dr. Broelsch received a call to return to his home region as the Professor and Chairman of the Department of Surgery at the University of Hamburg. He found this opportunity irresistible, and his success in Hamburg proved that you can go home again. However, his absence in North American Surgery and the University of Chicago is widely lamented as his world-wide reputation increases. It is a great personal pleasure to have my former colleague and dear friend, a true master surgeon, participate in *Surgical Practice Illustrated.*

The artist, Mr. Todd Buck, invited to illustrate Dr. Broelsch's superb techniques is new to this series and a very welcome addition. Mr. Buck received his B.A. at Iowa State University in the field of biological and medical illustration and then earned a Masters Degree in the Associated Medical Sciences at the University of Illinois at Chicago. His collaboration with Dr. Broelsch took place while both were residents of the Chicago area. Mr. Buck's work is marked by its clearness and accuracy in presenting difficult surgical procedures and biological subjects. He has a number of surgeons and physicians among his clients and has been invited to present work by a number of publishers including Churchill Livingstone and the Encyclopedia Britannica. He is a member of the Association of the Medical Illustrators and the Mid-West Medical Illustrator Professional Organizations. In 1991, he won the Award of Excellence for an illustrated college textbook granted by the Association of Medical Illustrators and has previously won several other awards for similiar achievements. It is a pleasure to include Mr. Buck amongst the distinguished artists participating in the *Surgical Practice Illustrated* series. I believe the reader will agree that his collaboration with Professor Broelsch has led to a highly valuable and unique publication for any student or physician interested in the diseases of the liver.

David B. Skinner, M.D.

Preface

Clinical application of advanced hepatic surgery has undergone a rapid expansion in recent years in response to improved knowledge of hepatic anatomy and physiology. Without consideration of the complex dual vascular supply, biliary drainage, and the circulatory requirements of the parenchyma, any hepatic operation can rapidly become a nightmare. Precise surgical technique, however, is still the key to successful liver surgery.

Through the epochal work of Dr. Thomas E. Starzl, liver transplantation has become the treatment of choice for end-stage liver disease. Intricate knowledge of the liver's anatomy has led to further innovative techniques in liver transplant surgery. Today, livers can be "tailor-made"—cut down to match the size of a young recipient. In this way liver lobes and segments are being transplanted as viable, independently functioning grafts. The improved results derived from utilizing segmental grafts from donors has reduced the "waiting-list mortality" for many children awaiting liver transplantation. The role of segmental transplantation has also been extended to include removing lobes from living donors.

In this book, I have attempted to provide a visual representation of the various procedures that can be performed on the liver. Many experts have described different techniques for any given situation dealing with hepatic surgery. A planned approach is emphasized for each procedure; the reader will discover a simple, clearly defined strategy that will enable him or her to perform the most complex operation. To meet individual needs, flexibility is strongly emphasized, and the consideration of abandoning a procedure should not be dismissed.

Every liver operation should begin with three considerations. First, is the lesion technically removable? Second, does the liver parenchyma allow for the removal of a certain mass of functional liver tissue? Third, can the procedure be performed safely?

Liver surgery has thrived as a subspecialty of general surgery because expertise is required, although surgery in this area often requires simultaneous resection of additional viscera in addition to a portion of the liver. Nevertheless, hepatopancreatobiliary surgery has evolved into an identifiable new field of surgical science and technique.

This book presents the basic principles of liver surgery applicable to surgeons with a particular interest in this field without placing undue reliance on additional technical devices, such as lasers, ultrasonic and water jet dissectors, and/or special clamps. These devices, although useful in certain situations, have added little to the proven value of parenchymal dissection through finger fracture or mosquito clamp techniques, which have withstood the test of time. There is no substitute for experience; it is one of the major determinants of the outcome of surgery. Hopefully, this book will clarify standards and limitations for surgeons performing liver surgery.

Christoph E. Broelsch, M.D.

Acknowledgments

I would like to acknowledge the outstanding work of Mr. Todd Buck, whose continuing observation in the operating room, combined with an excellent imagination and expert illustrations, has made this atlas possible.

I am indebted to Dr. David Lloyd for his editorial assistance and review of the manuscript and to Ms. Mary Burage, my secretary for many years at the University of Chicago Division of the Biological Sciences Pritzker School of Medicine, who was helpful in typing and reviewing the text.

Contents

Hepatic Resection

Hepatic resections consist of the removal of a lobe or segment of the liver, followed by subsequent regeneration of the residual parenchyma within a few weeks. Any malignant primary or secondary lesion of the liver requires removal to prevent further spread within the liver and elsewhere.

Identification and extension of a lesion require extensive work by ultrasonography, computed tomography (CT) scanning (with or without angiography in selected situations), celiac angiography, and hepatic venous outflow. Venography is required whenever resectability is in doubt. Percutaneous or laparoscopic biopsy is only indicated when surgery is seriously considered to be inadequate.

Radionuclide diagnostic technique has proven to be helpful in differentiating between various benign lesions. For instance, cavernous hemangiomas can definitely be diagnosed by trapping of ^{99m}Tc-labeled erythrocytes, focal nodular hyperplasias by absorbing ^{131}Iodine E-hida tracer into the hepatocytes. Benign lesions only prompt surgery by development of symptoms, signs of growth, possibility of malignant transformation, and spontaneous rupture.

Mortality of hepatic resection ranges between 0 to 15 percent, depending on the procedure to be performed, the underlying primary disease, and the functional status of the parenchyma. Identification of liver cell function is of utmost importance in preparing the procedure.

Any elevation of serum bilirubin significantly increases the risk of surgery to the extent that, prior to any resection or surgery of the liver, serum bilirubin should be either normal or normalized by stenting or external drainage. The jaundiced patient will *not* tolerate hepatic resections.

1 | *Various Types of Hepatic Resection*

A Hepatic anatomy is defined by its vascular structure. The portal vein and hepatic artery represent the afferent system to the liver; the efferent system consists of the hepatic veins draining into the inferior vena cava. Bile is excreted into the intestine via the biliary tree. Segmental bile ducts join to form two main hepatic ducts that combine to form the common hepatic duct, which receives the cystic duct, thereby becoming the common bile duct. This usually drains into the second part of the duodenum via the ampulla of Vater.

Although many variations are described, the vascular structures generally divide the liver into right and left lobes, the right comprising 60 percent of the liver mass and the left containing approximately 40 percent. A further subdivision into hepatic segments is based on anatomic principles defined by several authors, including Frerichs, Couinaud, and Starzl. For surgical purposes, however, the anatomic division of the two major hepatic lobes can be identified in a plane joining the gallbladder fossa to the inferior vena cava. Although part of the left lobe, the section of liver between the falciform ligament and the right lobe is termed the left median lobe or segment.

B Medial to the right lobe and lateral to the falciform ligament, the left median segment is removed when performing an extended right hepatectomy, which includes a right lobectomy and a left median segmentectomy. The left median segment is clearly a part of the left lobe, since it receives its blood supply from the left hepatic artery and the portal vein. Its venous drainage occurs through the left hepatic vein also. Seventy-five percent of the liver mass is removed through an extended right hepatectomy.

C A left lobectomy entails the removal of the caudate lobe, the left lateral segment, and the left median segment. However, the caudate lobe is occasionally left in place, despite the arterial and portal blood supply being disconnected, and will eventually atrophy.

D The left lateral segment represents only 25 percent of the liver mass and has its distinct individual portal and arterial blood supply. The latter often comes from the left gastric artery (17 to 23 percent). Biliary drainage is not uniform, although most of the segmental bile ducts join into a single left duct before merging with the left median duct and the caudate branch into the left hepatic duct. Note that several portal venous branches may enter the round ligament to supply the anterior portion of the left median segment. The line of dissection follows the falciform ligament until the left hepatic vein is identified. Arterial blood supply derives exclusively from an individual branch from the left hepatic artery, while portal venous branches show some variations.

E An extended left hepatectomy goes beyond the fossa of the gallbladder and includes the anterior portion of the median right lobe (Couinaud's segment 5) without compromising the venous outflow of the posterior segment. This is obviously performed for large tumors extending beyond the limits of the anatomic left lobe.

F Resection of the median left lobe is a preferred procedure for resection of isolated metastatic lesions in this region or for lesions comprising or compressing the confluence of the bile ducts. Because of the large bilateral surface of dissection, control of affluent and effluent vessels is imperative, as well as control of the integrity of the biliary excretion. Although it removes only a relatively small portion of the liver, this procedure is the most demanding of all liver resections.

G Removal of a segment of a lobe has become the preferred method of resection of isolated metastases. Individual segments can be removed with or without adjacent or additional resections while preserving sufficient tissue to maintain hepatic function. Peripheral segments can be removed this way, but care has to be taken not to compromise hepatic venous outflow, arterial circulation, and biliary drainage of the remaining liver.

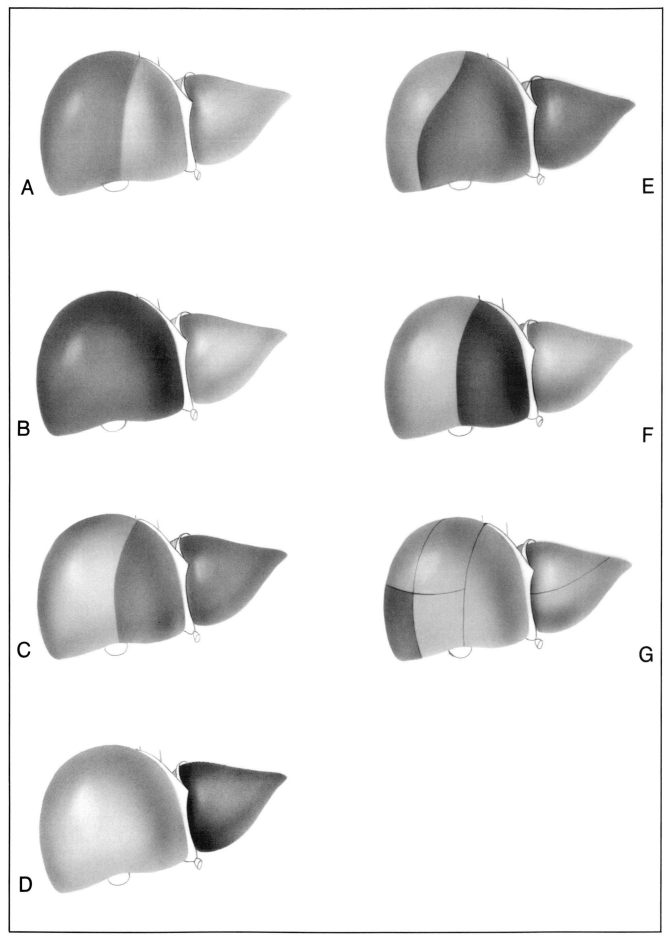

2 | *Patient Position and Surgical Incisions*

A

Most hepatic surgery does not require special patient positioning or arrangement, since thoracotomies are rarely performed and not usually anticipated. Supine positions with the right arm extended are preferred, with the abdomen slightly overstretched. Anesthetic setup is extremely important and must include endotracheal anesthesia, standard electrocardiographic monitoring, and a Swan-Ganz multilumen catheter, in addition to peripheral arterial monitoring lines and major anticubical infusion lines in both arms. Percutaneous oxygen detectors are helpful, and a Foley catheter is mandatory. The patient is laid on warming pads and both extremities wrapped in silver foil. The left arm is placed next to the body, isolated and wrapped for protection.

B
C

Laparotomies are performed through a bilateral subcostal and upper abdominal midline incision (Mercedes incision). Thorough palpation of the abdominal organs and the liver lesions is performed before the incision is extended onto either side. For a right hepatectomy, the incision is extended to the right midaxillary line to allow access to and control of the inferior vena cava below the liver.

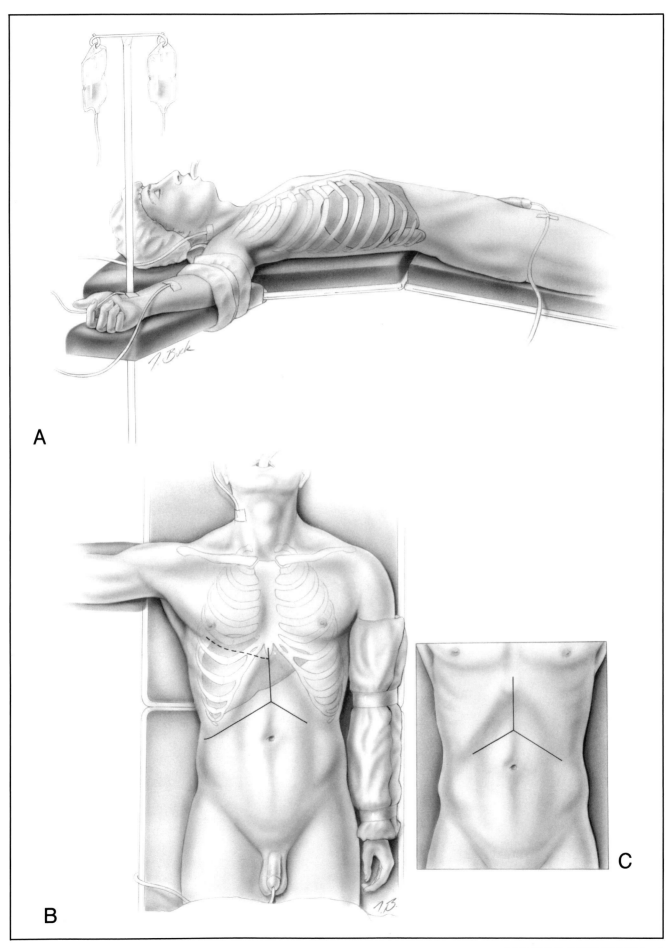

After laparotomy, retractors must be inserted to gain access to the liver. It is most important to use strong retractors, fixed to the operating table, to totally immobilize the operating field and lift the rib cage cranially. In females this is usually accomplished fairly easily, while males pose more of a problem. Should access be extremely poor, a thorocotomy through the seventh rib space could be considered; this can be performed on a patient in the supine position and may be indicated in cases of extensive diaphragmatic involvement with tumor.

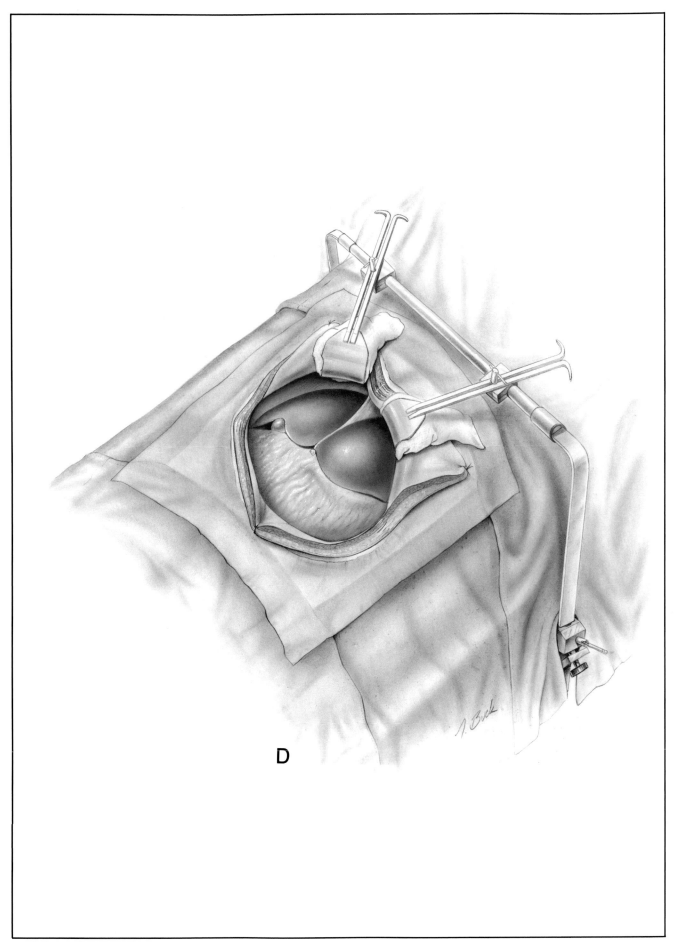

D

3 | *Right Hepatectomy*

A right hepatectomy removes all segments supplied by the right hepatic artery and portal vein. Control of the afferent and efferent vessels is of vital importance when performing this procedure, as total vascular control may be necessary. Control of bleeding from the surface by other means remains extremely difficult because of the mass of the tissue. Right hepatectomies carry a mortality risk of between 7 and 15 percent; intraoperative and postoperative bleeding may lead to a downhill spiral of complications, which in turn will lead to death, but liver failure or multisystem organ failure are usually the terminal events.

Mobilization of the right lobe and control of its vascular pedicles is of utmost importance. The round ligament is dissected from the anterior peritoneal layer. With a moistened lap pad, downward traction is placed on the liver to maintain tension in the falciform ligament, which is incised by electrocautery. Several vessels may need to be suture-ligated, depending on the degree of vascular collaterization, but this is not usually necessary in patients without portal hypertension. Usually, the thin falciform ligament can be easily divided. We would advise that the ligament be cut close to the abdominal surface, so that the majority of its tissue can be incorporated in mattress sutures for controlling bleeding at the cut surface of the liver.

Once the falciform ligament is completely divided, the dissection continues to the confluence of the hepatic veins, and then on to the right, dividing the right triangular ligament and freeing the dome of the right liver lobe completely. The small fissure between the right and left hepatic vein can be identified and a curved blunt clamp may be able to penetrate between the two vessels as they emerge from the liver. The left triangular ligament is not usually dissected because it may contain additional blood supply to the left lateral lobe. At this stage the tumor(s) can be assessed manually and with intraoperative ultrasound. The line of resection can be planned, preferably allowing a 2-cm tumor-free margin. Generally, resectability is determined by the involvement of hepatic veins or hepatic arteries, and not so much by portal venous anatomy. In cases where the tumor may involve the right hepatic vein and hepatic venous reconstruction may be indicated, a tourniquet must be placed around the suprahepatic vena cava to control bleeding, if necessary.

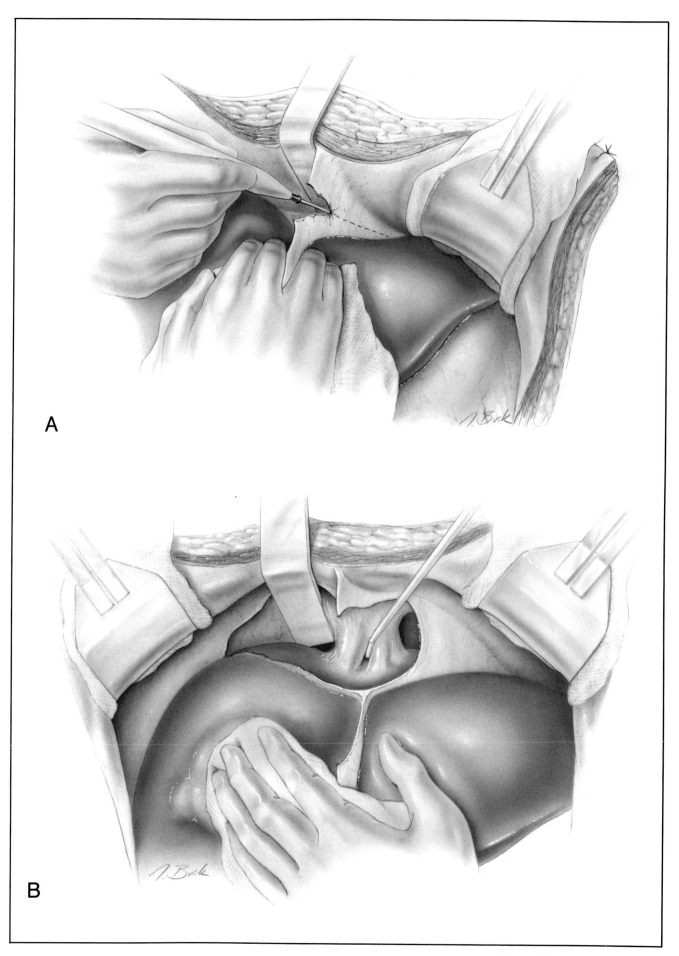

Mobilization of the right lobe continues with dissection of the right triangular ligament. The lobe is mobilized from its inferior peritoneal attachments, assisted by lifting the liver anteriorly and to the left. Most of the dissecting can be done with electrocautery, but some large diaphragmatic vessels should be suture-ligated. Strong retraction of the right rib cage and gentle pulling and rolling of the liver toward the left allows full exposure of the subdiaphragmatic space.

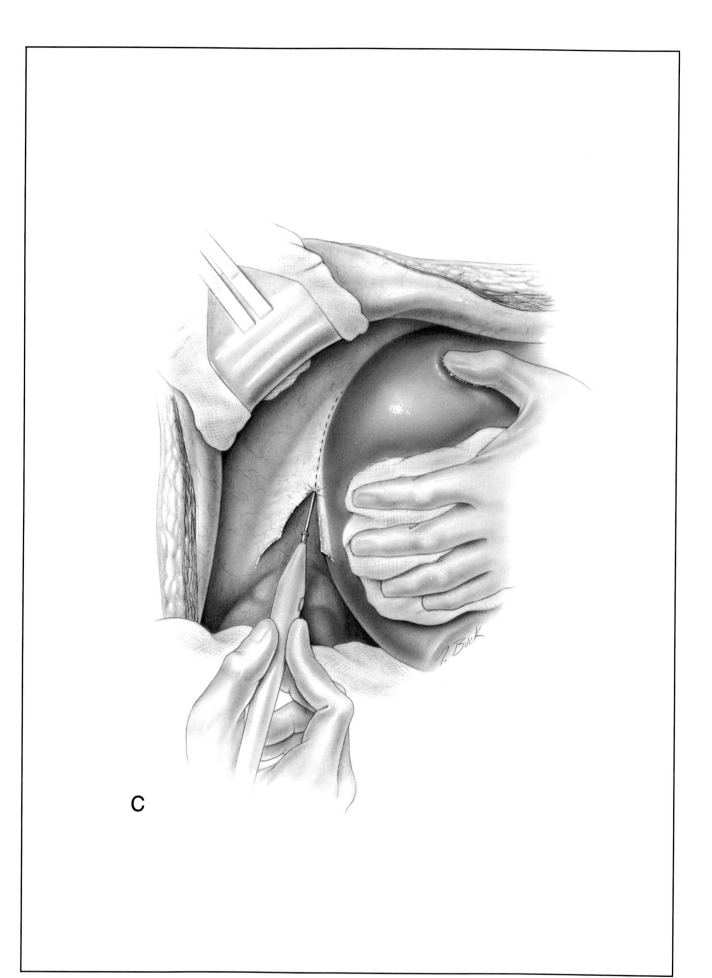

C

D Once the right lobe has been freed from its ligamental attachments, intraoperative ultrasound should be employed to further identify the limits of the lesion and its extension, as well as identifying other tumor sites within the whole of the liver. Tumor extension and vascular invasion should be assessed thoroughly, particularly in very large tumors, and careful attention must be paid to the venous anatomy.

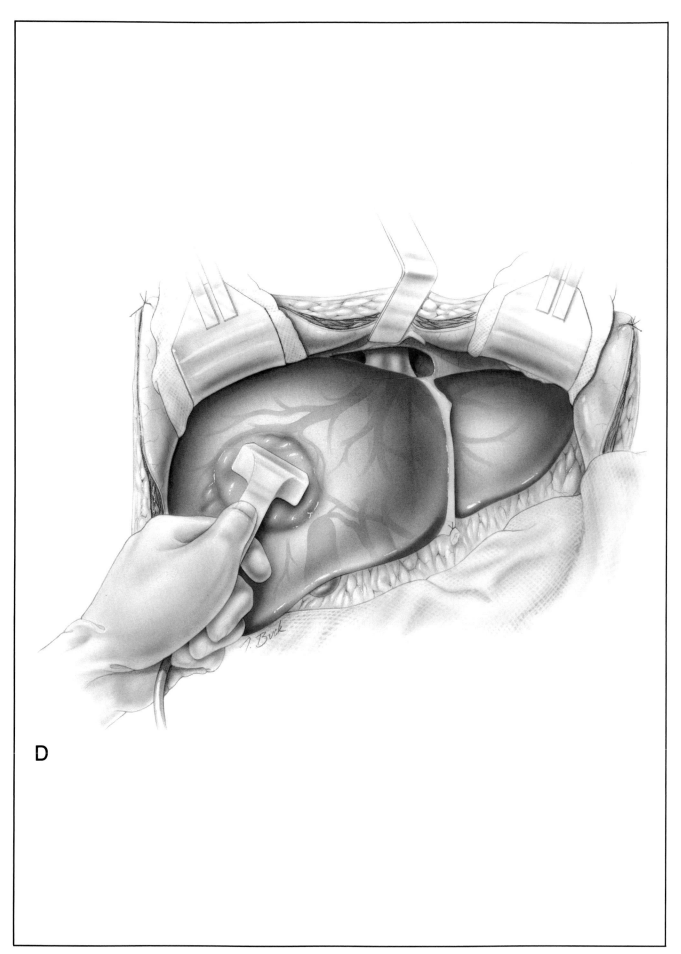

D

After the right lobe has been freed and resectability seems warranted, formal dissection of the hilum can commence. Calot's triangle is opened and both the cystic duct and artery divided between sutures. The hepatoduodenal ligament is palpated, not only to exclude portal nodal spread of tumor, but also to identify aberrant right hepatic arteries arising from the superior mesenteric artery.

Parallel to the common duct, the peritoneum is incised and the common hepatic artery is identified. No further dissection is necessary on the left side. The common duct is followed toward the liver.

The gallbladder is removed and the fossa of the gallbladder completely exposed. This allows better visualization of the right portal structures high up in the porta hepatis. Hemostasis is secured.

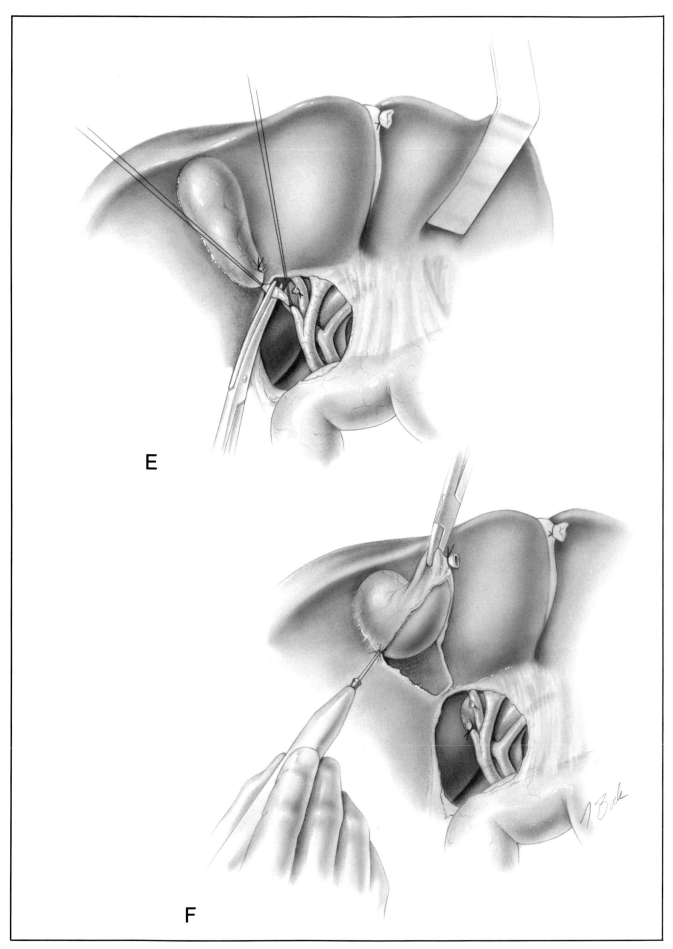

E

F

G The common hepatic duct is followed to the point of its penetration into the parenchyma. A thick layer of capsule and fibrous tissue marks the junction of the left and right hepatic duct. Approaching the duct from the right lateral position and preferentially from behind facilitates identification of the bifurcation. Note that the right hepatic artery usually dives beneath the right hepatic duct to enter the right lobe. This artery should be preserved as long as possible and tied extremely close to the parenchyma, because vascular supply of the common hepatic duct is mainly derived from the right hepatic artery. Once the bile duct junction is identified, a blunt curved clamp (e.g., an Overhaul clamp) is passed around the right branch of the hepatic duct. The duct is divided between two suture-ligatures. Gentle retraction of this duct allows the underlying right hepatic artery to be approached.

H The common hepatic duct is encircled by a rubber band and the right hepatic artery is identified and ligated close to the point of its penetration into the parenchyma. Double ligation secures the blind end of the right hepatic artery, and the dissection can continue to identify the right branch of the portal vein.

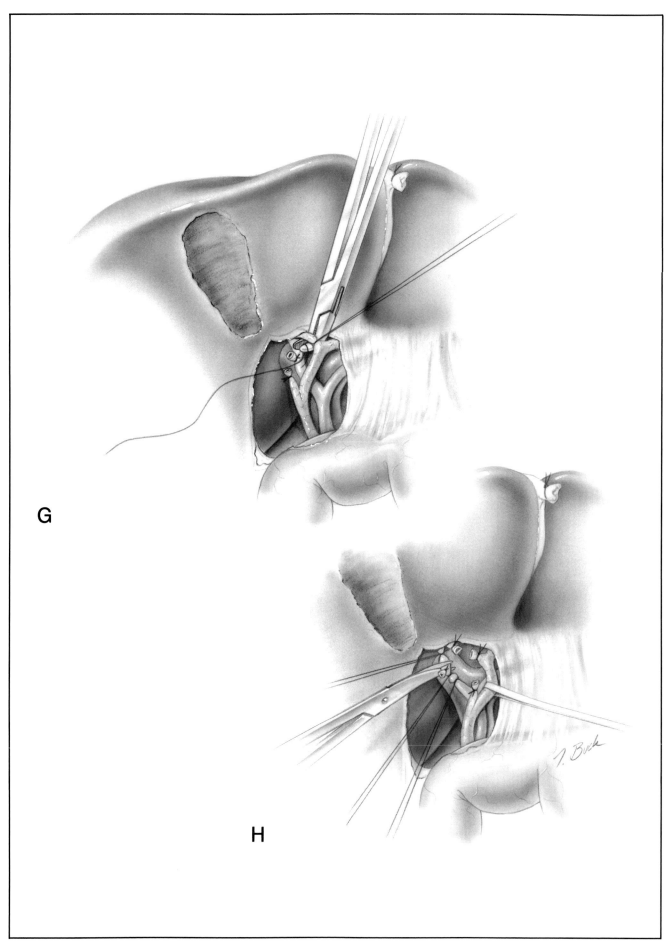

G

H

I The portal vein can be approached after the right hepatic artery has been divided and the common duct is retracted by a rubber band. The portal vein is identified using a combination of sharp dissection and blunt dissection with peanut-gauze (a swab at the tip of a Peau clamp [peanut-gauze dissector]). The bifurcation must be clearly identified and the right branch encircled with a curved vascular clamp. The portal vein is divided between curved vascular clamps, and the proximal end suture-ligated with a running monofilament suture. The distal end can be transfixed with a large suture. The clamps are removed.

Following disruption of the portal vein and the hepatic artery, an area of demarcation occurs that identifies the margin between the left lobe (i.e., left median lobe) and the right. The demarcation can be traced to the junction of the hepatic veins, and can be marked with electrocautery without penetrating into the parenchyma.

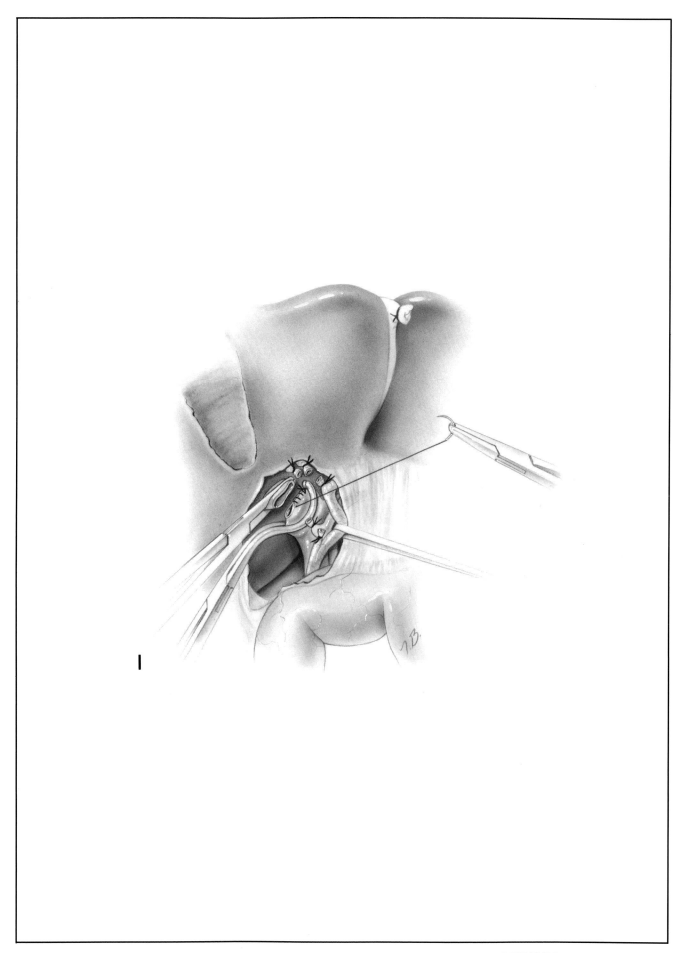

J A crucial part of a right hepatic lobectomy is the detachment of the right lobe from its hepatic vein as it enters the inferior vena cava. For a safer approach, the liver must first be cleared from the cava by suture-ligating all the accessory hepatic branches that lie on the lateral and anterior surfaces of the cava. Since the branches are relatively short and non-elastic, they should be encircled with a 3-0 suture and put on slight traction, allowing a small, curved vascular clamp to be placed on the caval end of the vein. The ligature is tied, and the vein can be safely divided.

K All venous branches on the caval side are suture-ligated with monofilament thread. Although the use of metal clips may speed up this dissection, some clips inevitably loosen and fall off, necessitating the use of additional suture-ligatures. We have abandoned using clips along the cava for this reason.

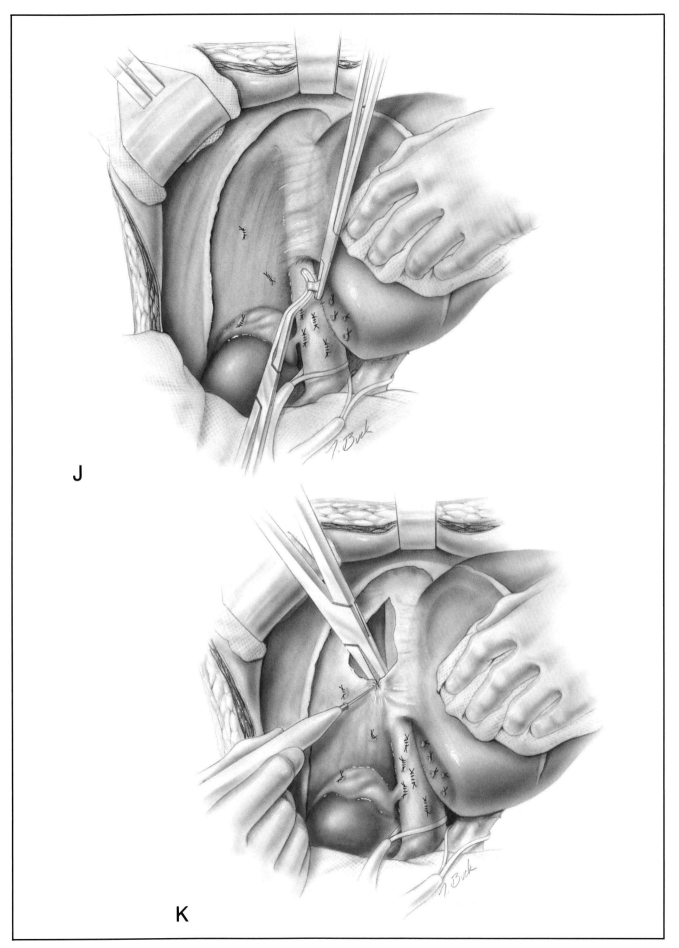

J

K

The dissection of the venous confluence around the entry of the right hepatic vein can be hazardous, and great caution is needed. There are frequently layers of peritoneum attaching the diaphragm to the liver capsule. These connections have to be dissected in a line parallel to the course of the inferior vena cava, with careful suture-ligation of the small branches of hepatic veins entering the proximal inferior vena cava. With the devascularized right liver lobe rolled over to the center, the right hepatic vein can be stretched out slightly, allowing a curved blunt clamp to encircle the large right hepatic vein without damaging the cava. This procedure should be done from above, but the exit site should always be visualized. This maneuver is usually the most difficult part of the operation, since any trauma to the hepatic vein can cause major bleeding, and full vascular occlusion of the liver is necessary. It may be prudent to inform the anesthesiologist during this maneuver, before there are any problems, so that the ventilation can be converted to a higher positive end-expiratory pressure ventilation (PEEP) in an attempt to avoid air embolism in case a vessel is opened.

 Once the right hepatic vein is encircled, a special curved vascular clamp is placed across it, clamping the base of the hepatic vein as well as part of the cava. The proximal end of the hepatic vein is suture-ligated with a 2-0 heavy suture. The caval end of the hepatic vein is closed with a continuous suture of 4-0 monofilament, without compromising the cava's lumen.

At the end of this step, the right lobe is totally devascularized and its resection can proceed along the line of vascular demarcation.

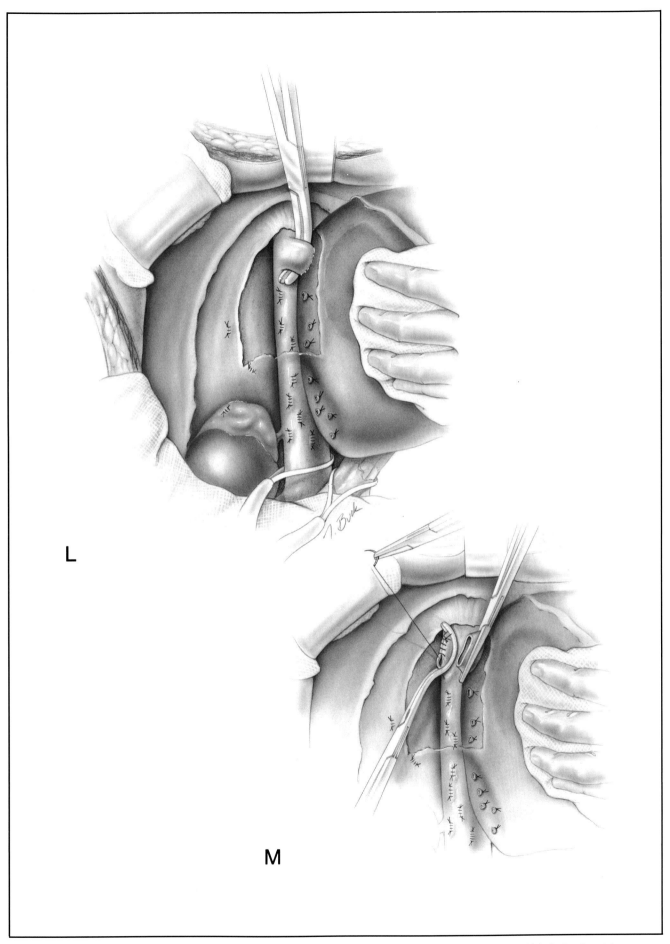

L

M

With the liver replaced to its normal position, the dissection of the parenchyma starts within the fossa of the gallbladder, following the line of demarcation. Practically, control of hemorrhage only needs to be maintained on the medial left side, where circulation is maintained. Electrocautery is used for incising the capsule and penetrating into the tissue. The mosquito clamp and fracture technique is used to identify the vascular and biliary structures within the crushed and dissected parenchyma.

In patients with normal liver function and an otherwise completely uneventful course during the operation, ligation of the hepatoduodenal ligament is preferred by tightening the tourniquet. This, of course, interrupts the portal and arterial blood supply to the left lobe of the liver also. Since the procedure of dissection is expected to last no longer than 15 to 20 minutes, including suture-ligation of the major branches at the cut surface, this maneuver saves time and prevents blood loss. Additional arterial branches from the left gastric artery, supplying the left lateral segment, are advantageous because occlusion of the hepatoduodenal ligament (Pringle's maneuver) can be extended safely up to one hour, since ischemia to the left lobe is avoided.

During this partial vascular exclusion, direct penetration into the parenchyma is performed. Clamps are placed on large ducts and vessels and mattress sutures, even without the use of clamps, used near the anterior part of the liver. Clamps are placed sequentially across the parenchyma and, when five or six clamps have been used, suture-ligated with mattress sutures.

With the hepatoduodenal ligament occluded, penetration into the parenchyma proceeds by suture-ligating the major structures, even on the side being discarded. The line of dissection stays close to the suture-ligated stumps of the right portal vein and right hepatic duct to preserve all structures supplying the left side, even if a small margin of devascularized tissue remains.

The disadvantage of partial devascularization by clamping only the hepatoduodenal ligament is that both sides of the dissection do not bleed, and some imagination and anatomic knowledge is needed to follow the anatomic border between the right and left lobe. The clear advantage is minimal blood loss and an extremely short time of devascularization.

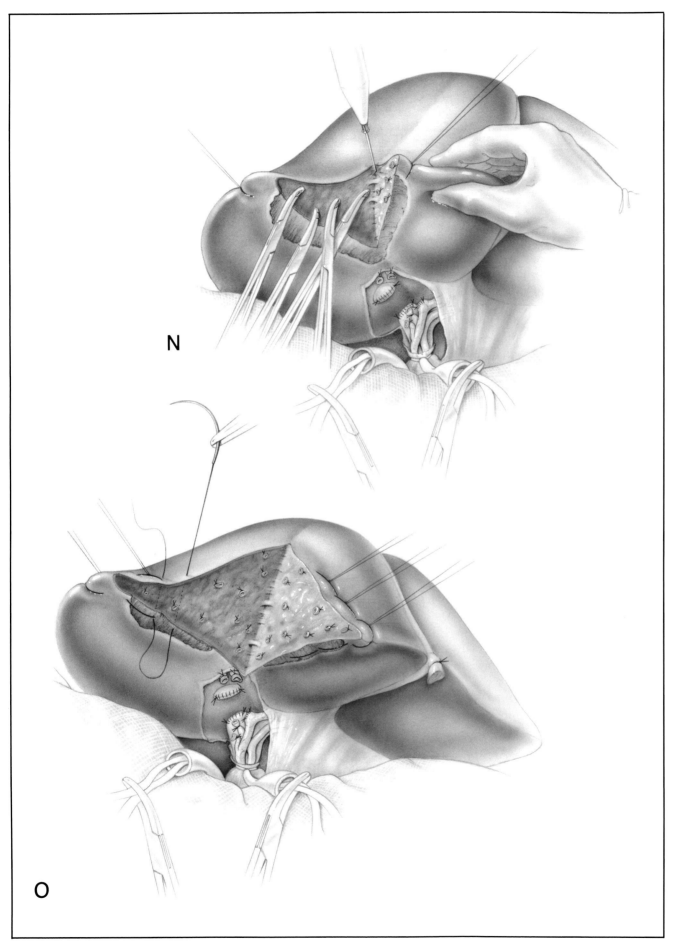

N

O

P An alternative method for dissection of the parenchyma is manual compression between thumb and index finger (sandwich technique), which requires skilled assistance. The hepatoduodenal ligament must be slinged, but does not necessarily need to be occluded. The index finger is placed parallel to the inferior vena cava and the thumb placed on the dome of the liver, just medial to the line of demarcation. While an assistant slightly compresses the tissue of the median left segment with the left hand, electrocautery can be performed with the right hand, while a second assistant aspirates blood and smoke. The surgeon uses clamps and scissors to penetrate the parenchyma, meticulously clamping the left side and clamping only the major vessels on the right side. The first assistant can demonstrate bleeding points to the surgeon by gradually releasing his sandwich-grip. These vessels are suture-ligated directly; in this way, blood loss is kept to a minimum.

Q During manual compression, the tissue is well-perfused and no devascularization is present, avoiding warm ischemia. Therefore, enough time is allowed for meticulous exposure of all vascular and biliary structures which can be individually suture-ligated. This is advantageous if there is slightly compromised liver function and damage to the left lobe must be avoided. The amount of blood that can be lost from the resection margin must not be underestimated—even on the right side—so all large veins should be ligated to minimize this blood loss.

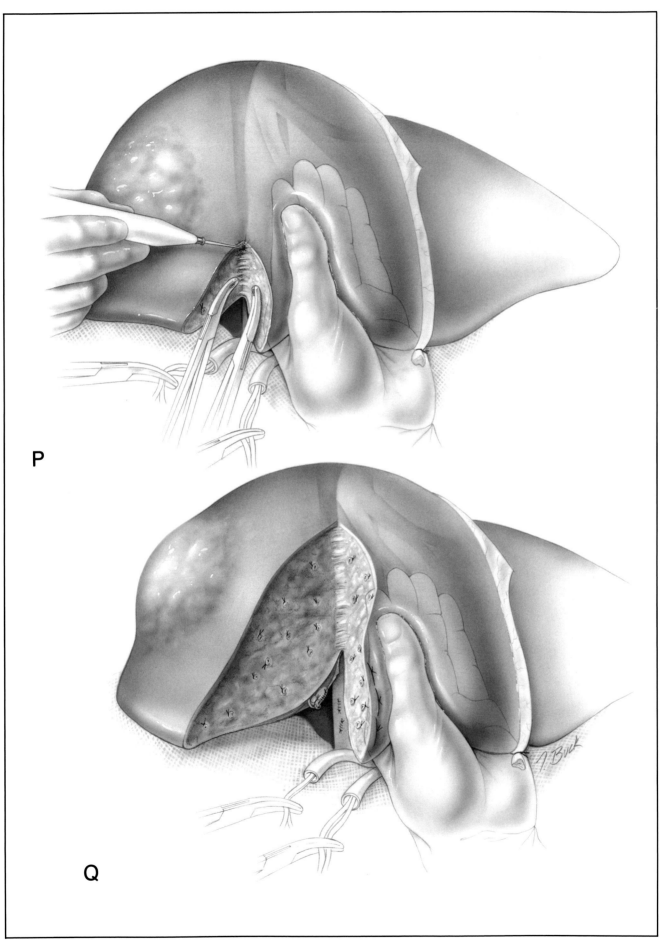

P

Q

Following complete removal of the right lobe, the resected surface of the left median lobe is carefully inspected. Suture-ligations are performed directly to control remaining bleeding points. Mattress sutures must be placed very close to the cut edge of the liver to avoid causing areas of devascularized tissue. Electrocautery, infrared light coagulation, or argon beam coagulation are occasionally employed to arrest minor oozing. Application of fibrin glue or the use of remnants of the falciform ligament or Gerota's fascia have also been advocated. However, meticulous technique during parenchymal dissection and surgical suture-ligation renders these other procedures superfluous, as they will not control surgical bleeding. All bleeding sites on the diaphragm and retroperitoneum must also be secured meticulously. Implantation of a flap of omentum is usually unnecessary, except for coverage of the cut surface, and usually the right flexure and the colon will ascend a little into the subdiaphragmatic space. Percutaneous drainage of this space before closure of the abdomen is mandatory. It must be remembered that, in 15 percent of all cases of hepatic right resections, thoracic drainage becomes necessary a few days following surgery. Thus, in cases where there has been extensive dissection of the diaphragm, particularly in reoperations of the right upper quadrant, it would be advisable to place a thoracic drain prophylactically.

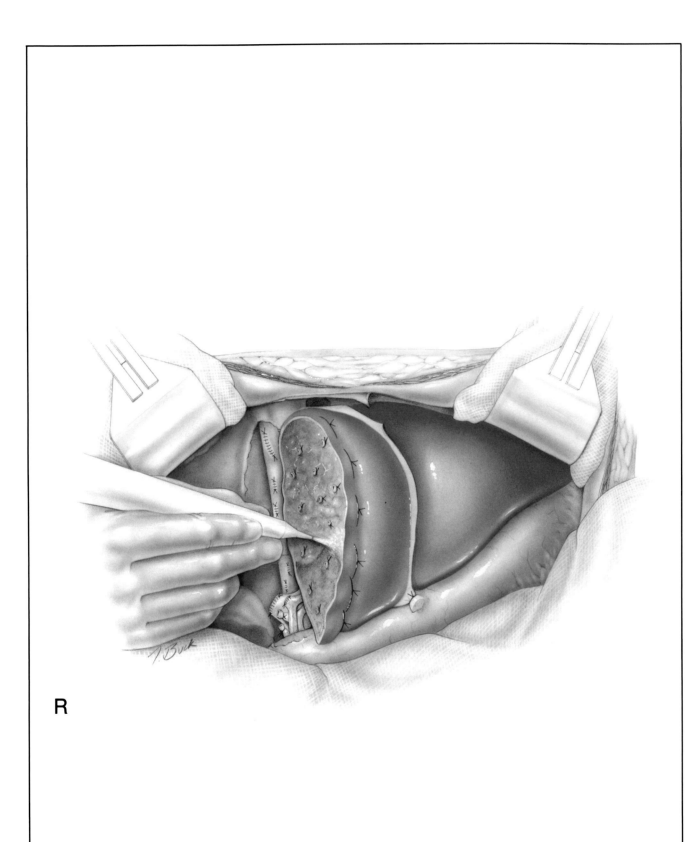

R

4 | *Left Hepatectomy*

A left hepatectomy includes the removal of the left lateral lobe and the left median segment (or lobe). The caudate lobe is part of the left lobe, but is usually not included in a standard left hepatectomy. However, the caudate lobe *should* be removed for malignant conditions involving the left lobe. Usually, the small bridge of liver tissue connecting the left lateral lobe with the caudate lobe can be easily disconnected, so that the caudate lobe can be left in place. Although it becomes disconnected from its arterial and portal venous blood supply, it may supply some degree of supporting hepatic function until it eventually atrophies. Removal of the caudate lobe includes careful disconnection of numerous small hepatic veins draining into the vena cava, since the lobe itself virtually embraces the inferior vena cava and can completely surround it.

When performing a formal left lobectomy, approximately 40 percent of the functional liver mass is removed. This usually does not present a risk of liver failure and many series are reported without mortality, particularly when the preoperative liver function is normal. Morbidity ranges between 5 to 10 percent, and includes biliary fistulas, necrotic margins and abscesses, hemoperitoneum, and pancreatitis. The cut surface of the right lobe presents a large area for potential bleeding and/or biliary leaks.

The patient is placed in a supine position and the abdomen is opened through a bilateral subcostal incision, with extension to the cephalad in the midline (Mercedes incision, see page 6). For this procedure, the subcostal incision to the left is slightly extended to obtain good exposure of the left lobe and the upper left triangular ligament. A standard cholecystectomy can be performed, but is not mandatory. The hilum is exposed and the dissection continues with a longitudinal incision of the peritoneum, medial to the common hepatic duct, to expose the left hepatic duct. Palpation of the hepatic artery usually identifies both its course and the location of its bifurcation. The left hepatic duct is identified, as well as the left portal venous branch, which is usually directly underneath the left hepatic bile duct.

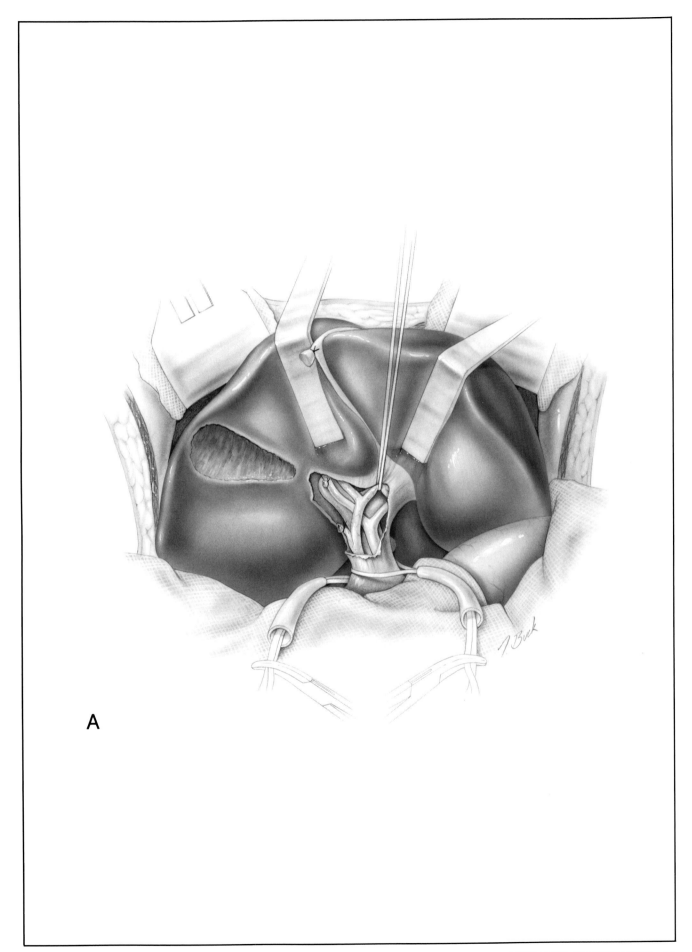

A

B Following careful identification of the confluence of the bile ducts, the left hepatic duct is disconnected and suture-ligated without compromising the lumen of the main hepatic duct. This act enables clear visualization of the bifurcation of the right and left hepatic artery. The left hepatic artery is ligated twice at its proximal end and once distally. It is then divided, allowing identification of the portal vein.

C After the left hepatic duct and left hepatic artery have been disconnected, the portal vein becomes easily accessible. The bifurcation of the right and left portal venous branch is identified and a special curved vascular clamp occludes the proximal end of the left portal vein. The portal vein is then divided and both ends are suture-ligated with running 5-0 monofilament suture to prevent obstruction at the proximal part. By staying close to the bifurcation, a branch supplying the caudate lobe can occasionally be preserved if the caudate lobe is not included in the left hepatectomy procedure.

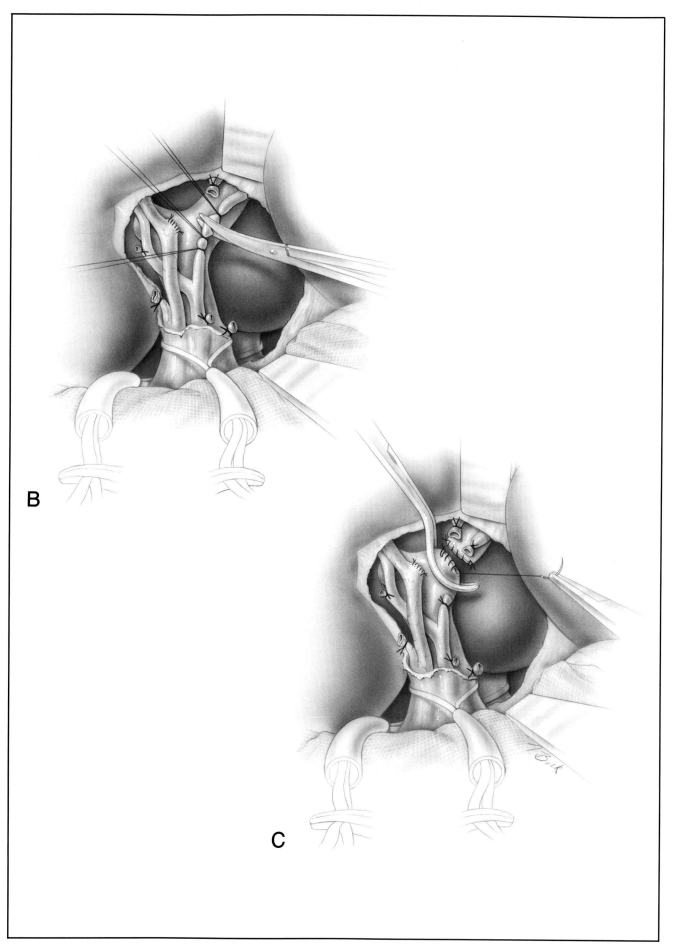

B

C

*D*once dissection of the hilum of the liver has been completed, vascular demarcation of the left lobe identifies the line of resection. The falciform ligament is divided by electrocautery to the bifurcation of the right and left hepatic veins. It is important to continue the dissection right onto the surface of the sub-diaphragmatic inferior vena cava in order to identify the orifices of both the left and right hepatic veins. Usually there is a fibrous rim that can be explored with a specially curved clamp, without penetrating either into the hepatic parenchyma or into the inferior vena cava.

The triangular ligament to the left is dissected by electrocautery, and the left lateral lobe is completely mobilized. Careful attention is paid to small branches coming from the diaphragm and entering the capsule of the liver. Substantial bleeding can occur from these vessels, and they often require suture-ligation for control. Occasionally, the lateral tip of the left lobe is adherent to the capsule of the spleen, and too rigorous a retraction may cause a splenic capsular tear, necessitating splenectomy.

Usually, the lobe can be freed easily and rolled over toward the right side to allow visualization of the caudate lobe and the lesser omentum. The lesser omentum is also dissected by electrocautery. In about 20 to 27 percent, a separate left hepatic artery can be identified, originating from the left gastric artery. Dissection and suture ligations are obviously required.

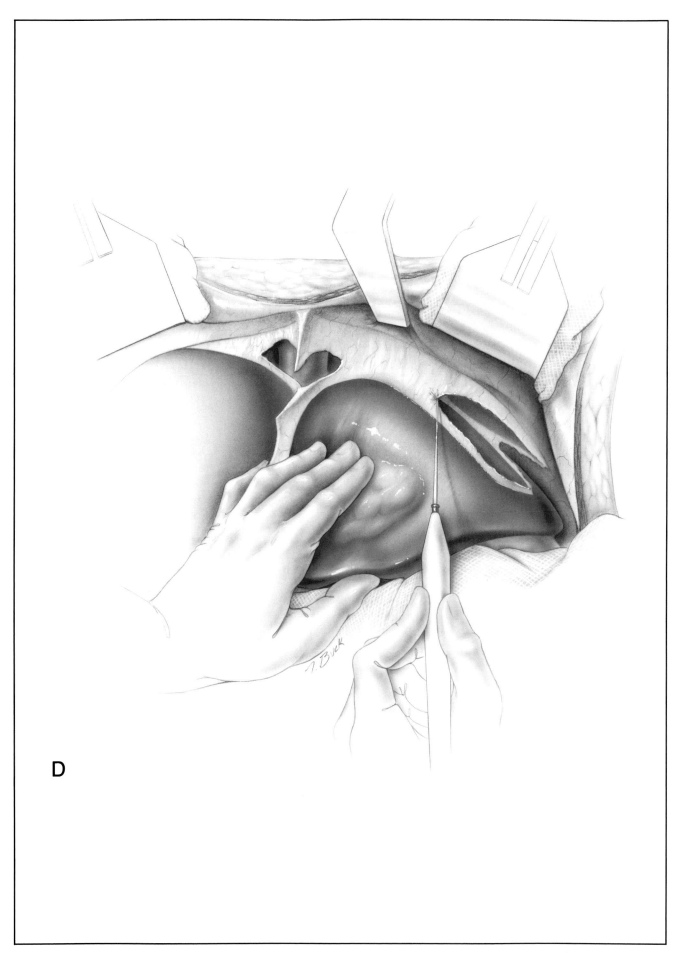

D

With the left lateral lobe pulled over to the right lateral side, the bridge of tissue connecting the caudate lobe, the parenchyma of the left lateral lobe, and the left median segment must be separated. This is done by mosquito clamp and fracture techniques, with careful attention paid to the small branches entering the inferior vena cava, which must be carefully suture-ligated. During this procedure, it is usually possible to identify a small bile duct arising from the caudate lobe; this is suture-ligated.

Since the hilar structures are already dissected, a gentle approach into the parenchyma can continue lateral to the left hepatic duct and the left hepatic artery. The line of demarcation is usually clearly visible even from the posterior surface of the left lobe. The advantage of this approach is that the left hepatic vein can be identified. A special curved clamp is introduced into the fissure between the left and the right hepatic veins. Its tip should lie directly on the cava and point to the left and medial direction. By approaching from the posterior surface, this tip of the clamp serves as a target and allows penetration of the tissue without running the risk of traumatizing the median and left lateral hepatic vein.

With the left lobe gently pulled to the right lateral side, the left hepatic vein can be safely clamped with a special curved vascular clamp. A straight clamp can be used to occlude the central portion of the hepatic vein.

With both clamps in place, the left hepatic veins are suture-ligated without compromising the caval diameter. During this procedure the anesthesiologist may want to exert slight PEEP, to prevent air embolism in case the clamp on the inferior vena cava orifice should slip.

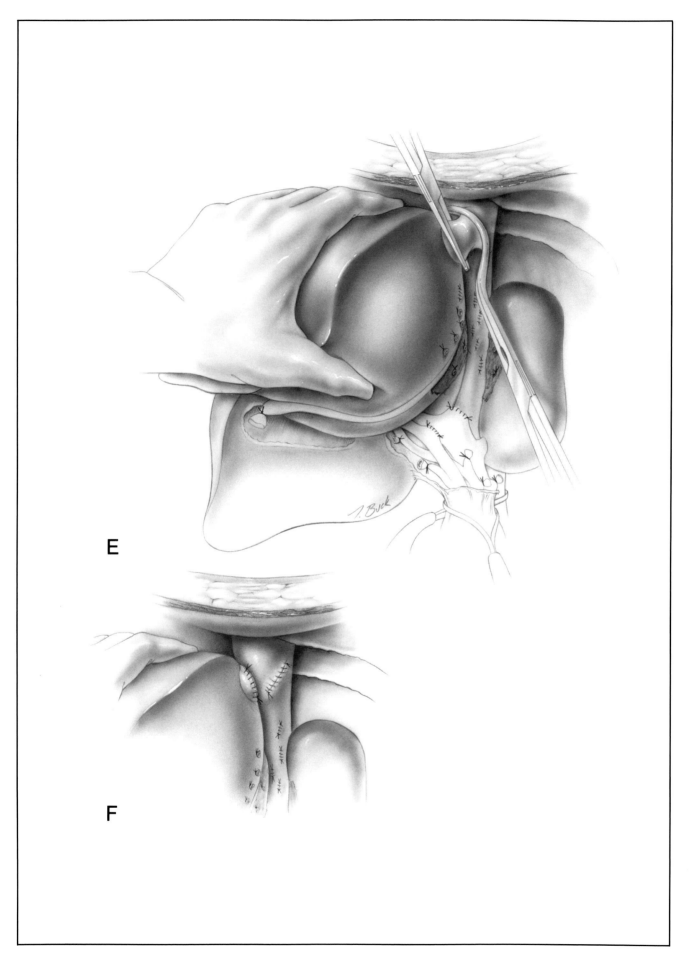

E

F

G Dissection of the parenchyma starts exactly at the line of vascular demarcation in the fossa of the gallbladder. With electrocautery leading the way through the parenchyma, mosquito clamps are applied to secure vessels on both sides, particularly on the remaining right side of the liver. With the hilar structures identified and disconnected, and the hepatic veins disconnected as well, the left lobe is rendered virtually avascular. The line of dissection is apparent, since disconnection of the posterior surface has already prevented bleeding from the inferior vena cava. Thus, dissection can be performed swiftly and bleeding is only encountered from the right side.

H Tightening the tourniquet around the hepatoduodenal ligament allows for amputation of the left lobe within a few minutes without undue blood loss. In contrast, only bleeding from the right side has to be controlled, which can be done by isolated clamping of vascular structures at the surface and subsequent suture-ligations. Only a small amount of attention has to be given to the left lobe, perhaps by using well-placed mattress sutures to prevent residual bleeding from the left lobe; this allows for virtually no blood loss during the entire procedure.

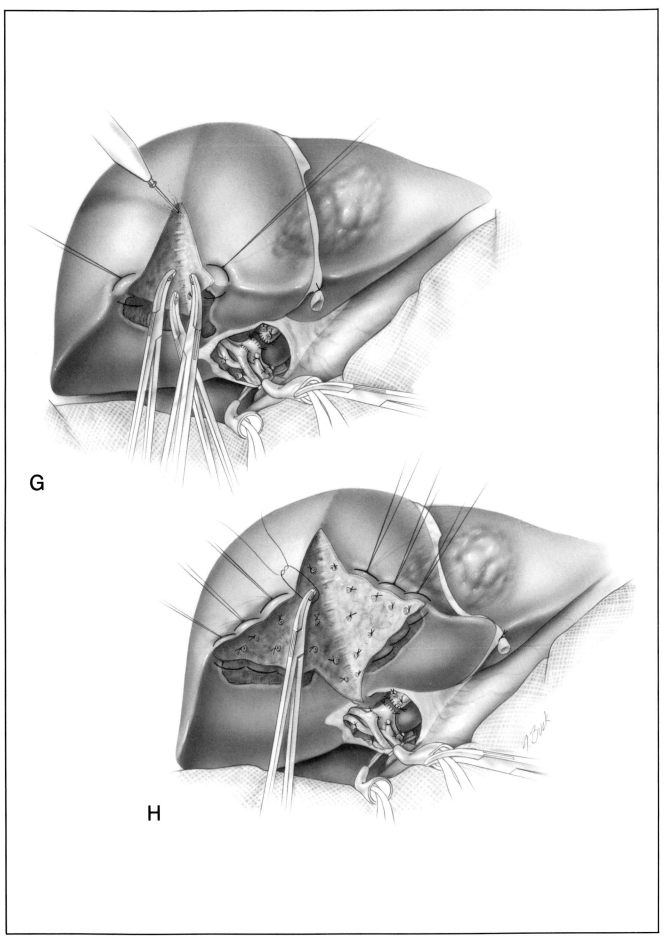

G

H

I The ultimate method for dissecting the devascularized parenchyma of the left lobe without clamping the hepatoduodenal ligament or the inferior vena cava includes a slight bimanual compression of the margin of the right lobe by the assistant, while the surgeon continues to dissect the parenchyma with electrocautery. Clamps are carefully placed to avoid bleeding from the cut edge of the right lobe.

With the posterior surface of the left lobe dissected, the index finger of the assistant can compress the parenchyma posteriorly, while the thumb, on the anterior surface, exerts counterpressure to prevent major bleeding.

J Without clamping of the hilar structures, the dissection follows the line of demarcation, allowing for deep penetration into the parenchyma. During this step, the liver is left in its normal anatomic position. With the bimanual compression, the assistant reveals the vital structures of the hilum and the hepatic venous outflow to the surgeon, allowing safe amputation of the left lobe. Proceeding this way, there is almost no danger of penetrating into the vital branch of the right portal vein or compromising the right hepatic venous outflow.

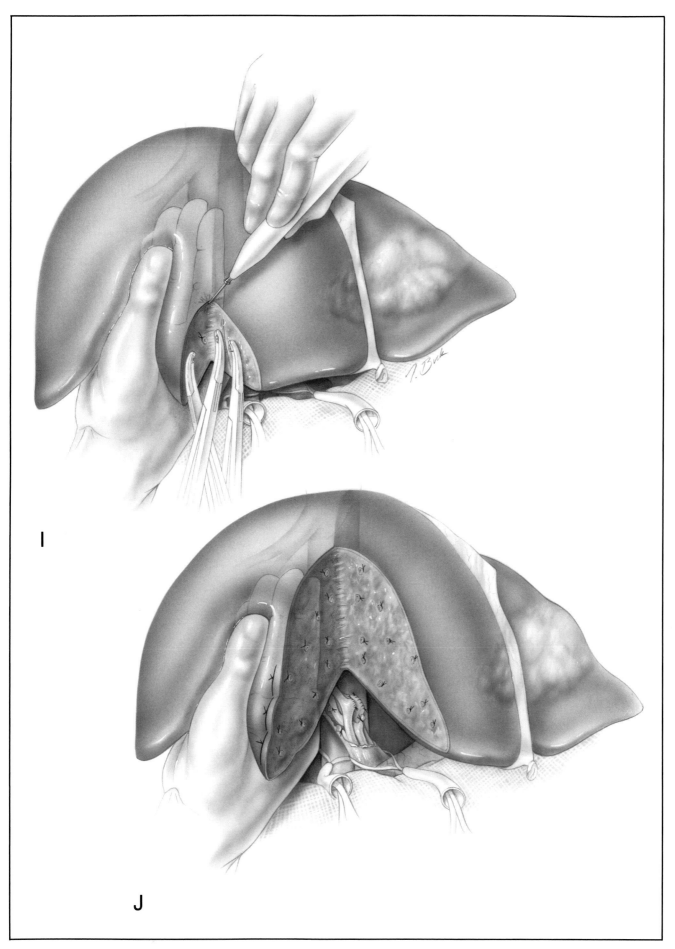

I

J

Once the procedure is completed, the dissected surface area can be reduced by placing a line of mattress sutures along the cut edge. Sutures must not be placed too deeply into the liver; otherwise, necrosis and/or abscess formation results. Major vessels require careful, isolated suture-ligation. Closure of the lesser sac is not required. Continual bleeding points must be secured surgically, although minor surface oozing may be controlled by using an argon beam coagulator, infrared light coagulator, or fibrin glue. Draining the raw surface is mandatory, as bleeding and bile leakage occur frequently. Finally, the patency of the hepatic artery is confirmed and the stump of the left hepatic duct is re-examined to confirm secure ligation.

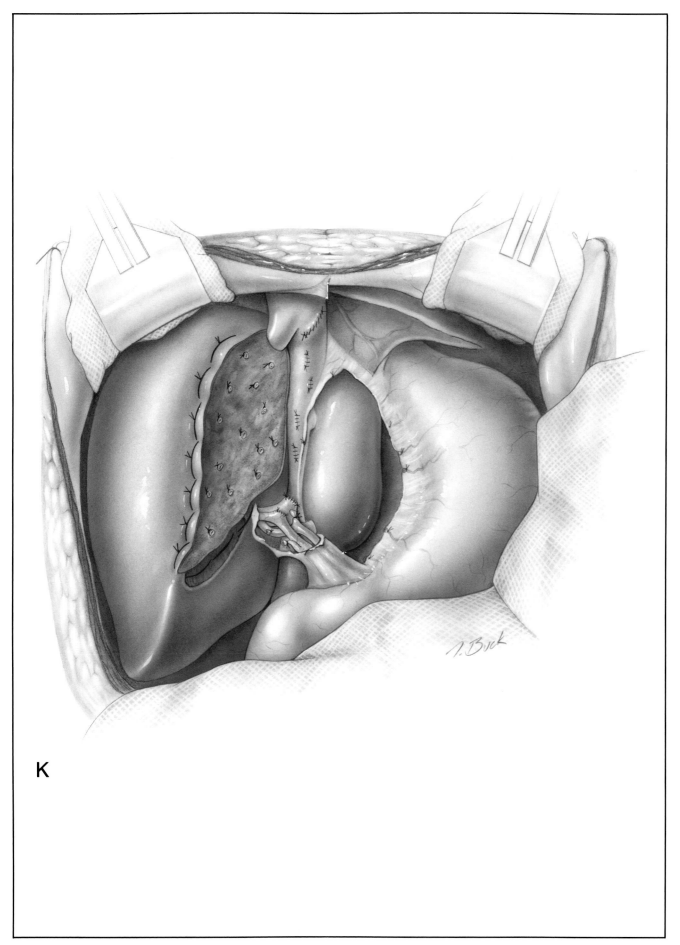

K

5 | *Left Hepatectomy Including Removal of the Caudate Lobe*

Removal of the caudate lobe adds a significant technical factor to the left hepatectomy procedure. This procedure is indicated whenever tumor tissue extends into the caudate lobe or the caudate lobe is involved in metastatic disease. Involvement of the caudate lobe may signify obstruction of the infrahepatic cava and, perhaps, hepatic venous involvement. Therefore, clarification regarding resectability must be obtained either preoperatively by venography, or intraoperatively by use of ultrasound.

A The beginning of the procedure follows the technique described for left hepatectomy, with isolation of the hilar structures and disconnection of the falciform ligament and the left triangular ligament. The lesser omentum is dissected and the caudate lobe visualized. A tourniquet is placed around the infrahepatic inferior vena cava, and the caudate lobe is subsequently freed of its hepatic venous connections. Mobilization is facilitated either by retractors or by the hand of the assistant, which allows for visualization of each single heptic venous branch and careful suture-ligation. Occasionally, the caudate lobe extends far to the posterior side of the inferior vena cava and contains hepatic venous branches of substantial size and diameter. These need to be occluded with vascular clamps and suture-ligated.

B With the caudate lobe freed of its hepatic venous attachments, the posterior surface of the left lobe of the liver can be explored and disconnected from the rest of the inferior vena cava. At the same time, visualization of the left hepatic vein is facilitated. It can then be isolated and divided as described above. The procedure is completed by following the routine description of a left hepatectomy, disconnecting the parenchyma either by occlusion of the hepatoduodenal ligament or by bimanual compression of the surface of the remaining right lobe.

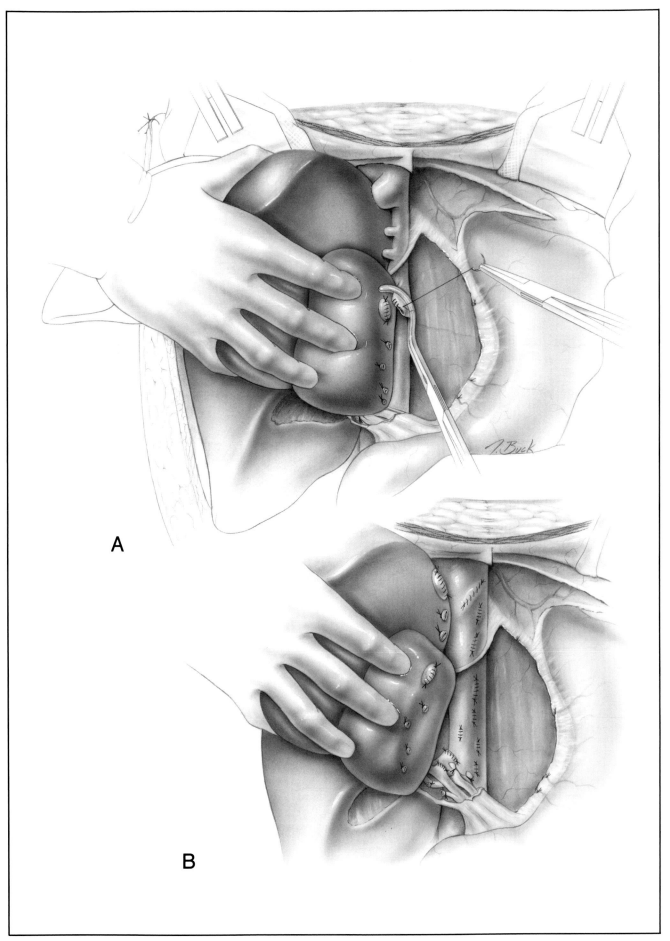

A

B

6 | *Left Hepatectomy Including Reconstruction of the Inferior Vena Cava*

The need for this procedure is rarely encountered, but is described here because, occasionally, hepatic resections can be extended into settings where parts of the inferior vena cava are involved, or when malignant tumors are located between the left lateral lobe and the caudate lobe. With a tumor in such a central location, the portal vein is often thrombosed. However, when the tumor is easily palpable and does not invade beyond the caudate lobe into the retroperitoneum or onto the lesser curvature of the stomach, resection is feasible. Intraoperative ultrasound will help to confirm the involvement of the hepatic and portal veins, which would preclude resection. These veins must not be involved.

With the tumor located to the left side, the procedure is approached as for a left hepatectomy. In this case, dissection of the falciform ligament, the triangular ligament, and the lesser omentum precedes any dissection of the hilum of the liver. If the hilum itself is free of tumor, the dissection is carried out as for a left hepatectomy. Once this is completed, the hilar structures are gently pulled over to the right lateral side to expose the cava. Tourniquets are placed around the cava, as well as the hepatoduodenal ligament.

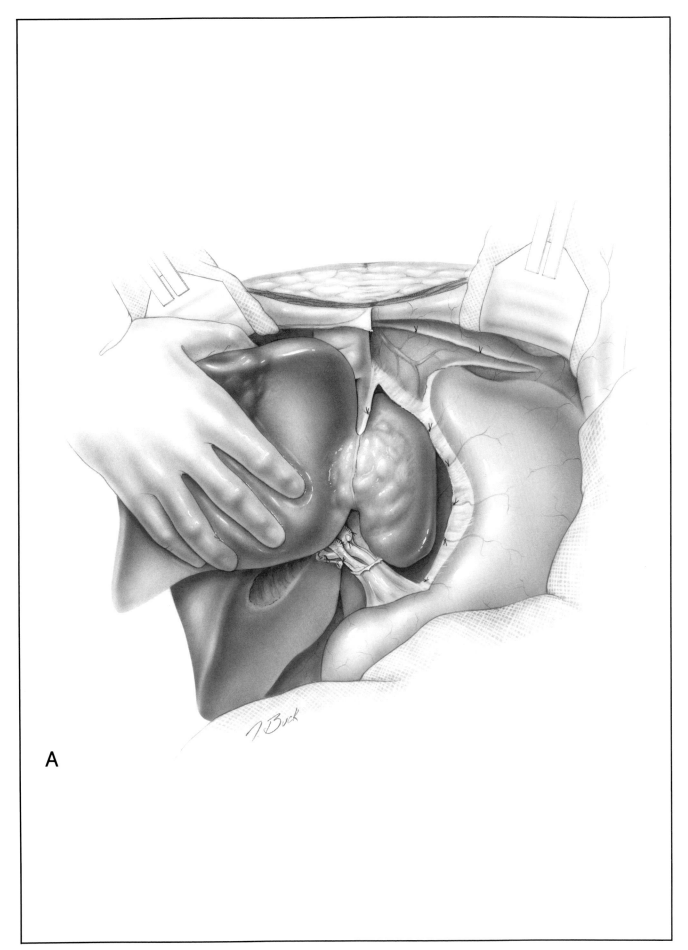

A

In order to facilitate isolation of the inferior vena cava at the site of penetration of the tumor from the caudate lobe, the right lobe of the liver needs to be mobilized as well. This is performed by the dissection of the right triangular ligament with electrocautery. Here, several diaphragmatic branches need to be suture-ligated until the right lobe can be rolled over gently to the left medial site, exposing the right lateral margin of the infrahepatic vena cava. Beginning from the right side, the adrenal vein and small hepatic venous branches coming from the right lobe to the vena cava are suture-ligated.

Gradually, the posterior surface of the right lobe is exposed. Branches from the right hepatic lobe entering the inferior vena cava are suture-ligated, with careful preservation of the main right hepatic vein. This posterior approach allows for full control of the cava above and below the tumor.

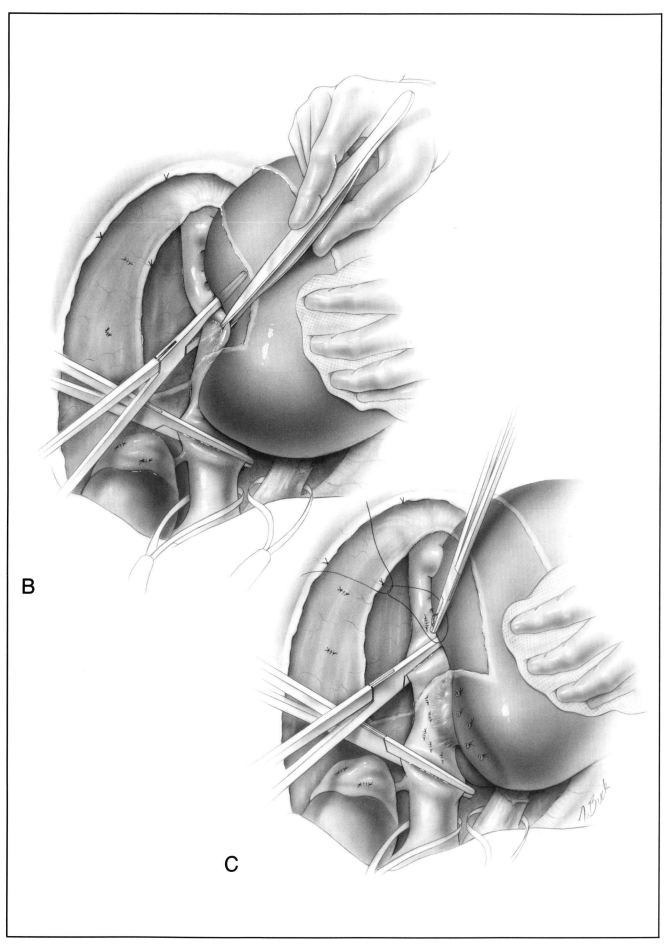

B

C

D The dissection continues with the liver gently rolled over to the right lateral side, exposing the left hepatic veins, which are then formally clamped and suture-ligated, allowing futher exposure of the posterior surface. The caudate lobe is mobilized by dissection of the retroperitoneum, leaving an adequate tumor-free margin. Careful attention must be paid to lumbar branches.

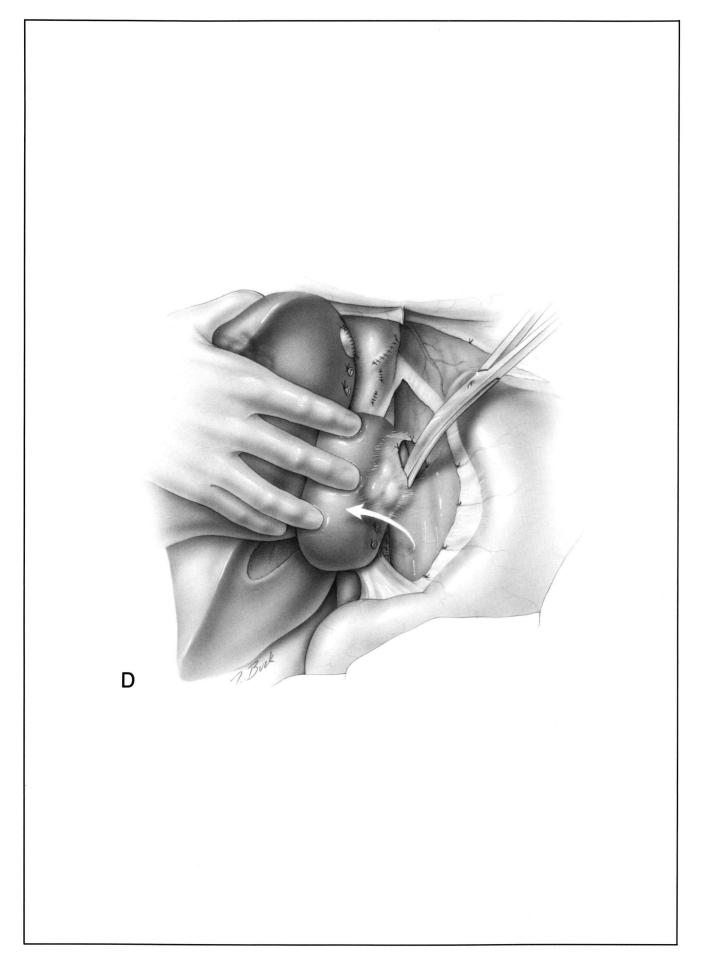

D

E The caudate lobe is disconnected from the retroperitoneum entirely, and is now attached only to the anterior wall of the cava. The hilar structures have been dissected as for a left hepatectomy and the hepatic veins have been suture-ligated. The left lobe is entirely devascularized and fully mobilized. At this point, cross-clamping of the cava must be performed.

F The wall of the inferior vena cava is excised en bloc with the tumor in the caudate lobe. Posterior lumbar vessels not previously ligated must be underrun from inside the cava with 6-0 monofilament suture.

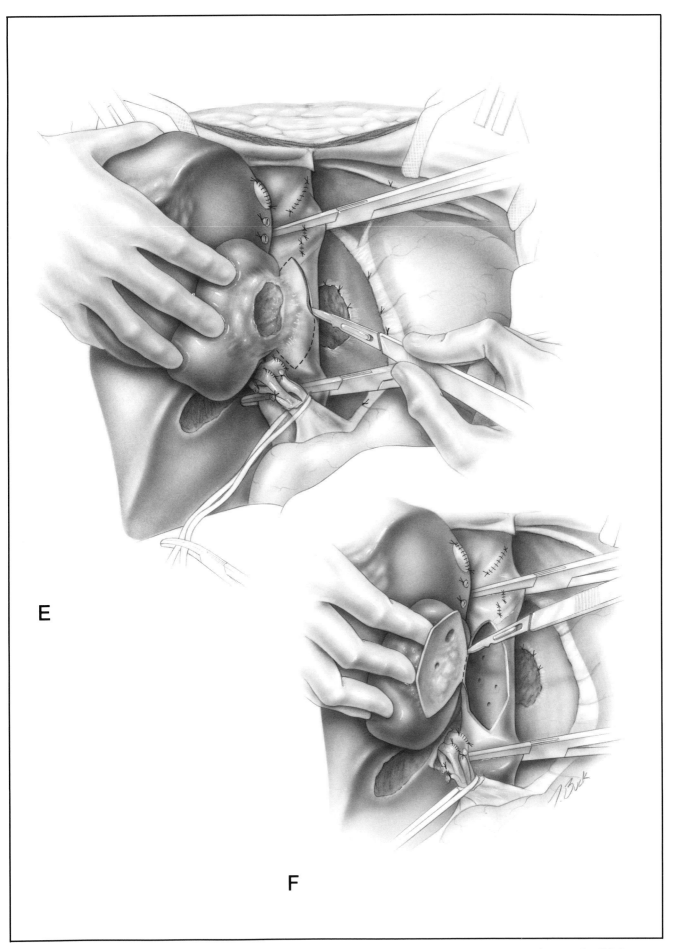

E

F

During this cross-clamping procedure, the devascularized left lobe can be disconnected completely from the remaining right lobe. For this approach, the hepatoduodenal ligament may be safely occluded with a tourniquet. The procedure follows the line of anatomic devascularization and is usually performed without major blood loss (see pages 39–41).

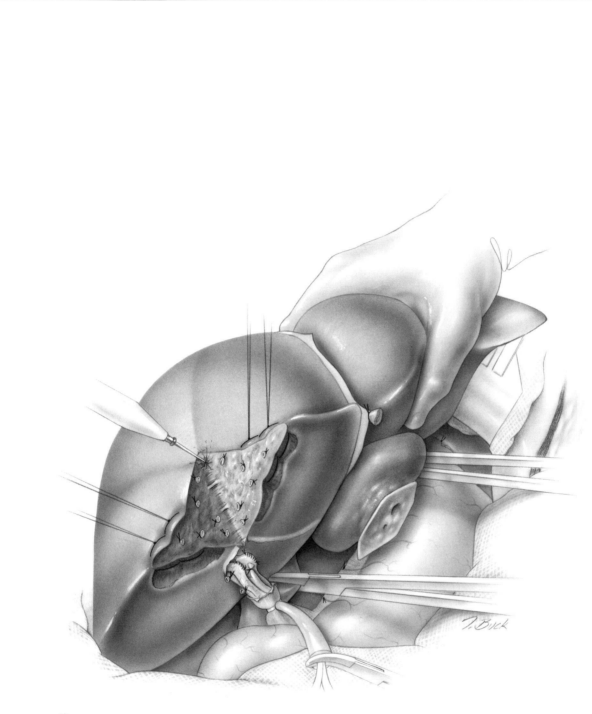

G

Once the left hepatectomy is completed, bleeding sites on the cut surface of the right lobe are controlled. A line of mattress sutures are placed along the cut edge, and the portal and arterial blood supply to the right lobe can be restored. The operating site must be rendered hemostatically dry; remaining lumbar veins are underrun.

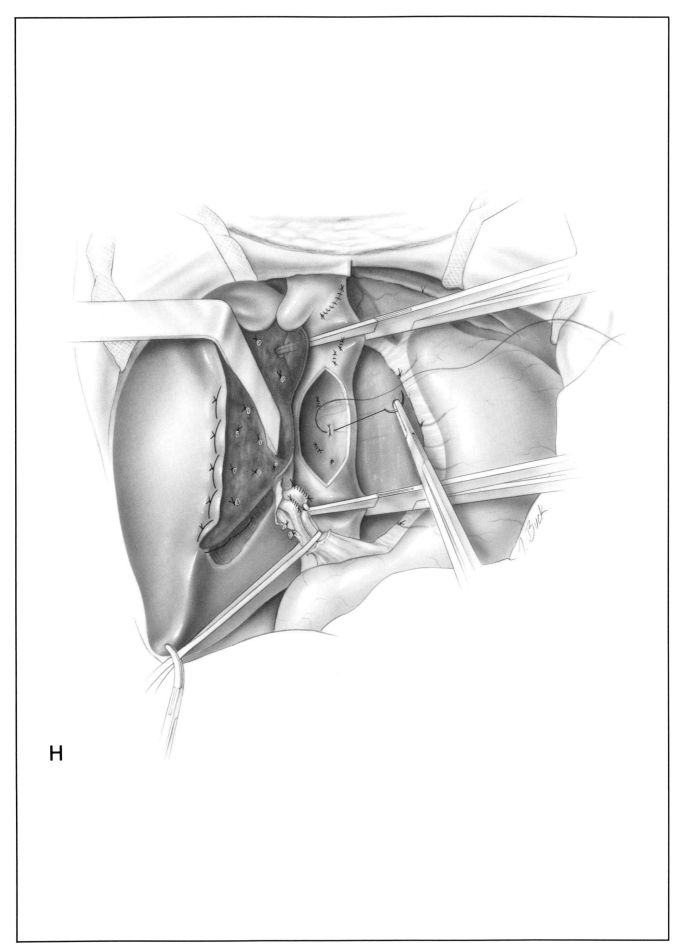

H

I   To repair the large defect in the inferior vena cava, an autologous venous graft is prepared from the patient's saphenous vein.

J   To increase the diameter of the graft enough to close the defect without causing stenosis, the graft is opened longitudinally and cut in half.

K

L   The two halves are sewn together using continuous 5-0 monofilament suture, and the corners are tailored to match the shape of the defect.

    The defect in the inferior vena cava is now reconstructed with the patch, using 5-0 monofilament continuous sutures. Before the final closure, the lower caval clamp is released slightly to allow the release of air bubbles and prevent air emboli.

    The reconstruction is completed and the caval clamps removed. Alternatively, a Gore-Tex prosthesis or prepared cadaveric vein patches could be used.

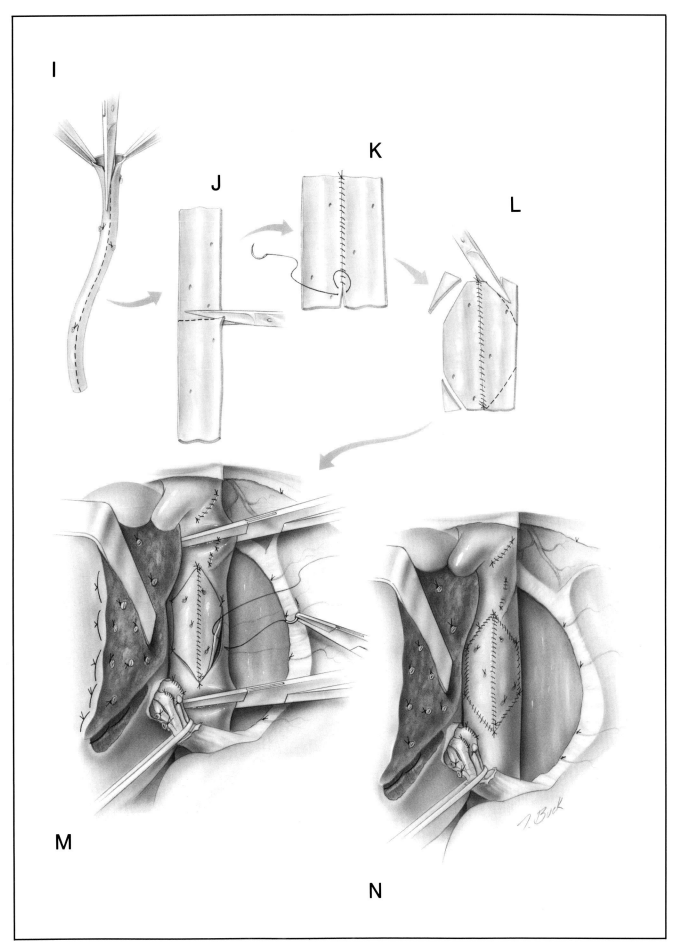

I

J

K

L

M

N

7 | *Extended Right Hepatectomy*

Extended right hepatectomy includes the removal of the entire right lobe of the liver and, additionally, the removal of the left median segment (Couinaud's segment 4). The operation incorporates the largest possible reduction of liver tissue, removing approximately 75 percent of functional liver mass. But, whenever a lesion in the right lobe, extending to the median left segment, has grown to the size that a right extended hepatectomy is indicated, compensatory regeneration of the left lateral lobe has occurred, so that, in actuality, less than 75 percent of functional liver mass is removed. The size of the left lateral lobe becomes a prognostic parameter, since a small left lateral lobe will not be able to maintain normal liver function if significant functioning liver tissue is removed with the right tumor; liver failure undoubtedly ensues. It is for that reason that, before any extended right hepatectomy is performed, liver function should be normal and ischemic liver damage to the left lateral lobe avoided under all circumstances.

Situations requiring a right extended hepatectomy are usually large primary liver tumors or multilocular metastatic liver disease. Apart from assessing the tumor with computed tomography (CT) and contrast-enhanced scans, celiac angiography is mandatory in ascertaining patency of the left branch of the portal vein. Portal venous thrombosis is a contraindication for any major partial hepatectomy, although, technically, the patency and flow of the portal vein could be restored. The patency of the hepatic artery must also be confirmed preoperatively by celiac angiography. Centrally located lesions involving the left hepatic artery as well as the right also render the procedure technically impossible. In addition, cholestasis presents a contraindication for this major procedure because of impaired excretory liver cell function and impaired liver regeneration.

The absence of vascular involvement and the extent of the tumor or presence of additional metastases are confirmed by intraoperative manual assessment and the use of intraoperative ultrasound. In particular, the patency of the left lateral hepatic vein, the portal vein, and the inferior vena cava can be confirmed.

With the right lobe of the liver completely freed from its ligamenta and vascular attachments, the index finger of the surgeon is placed on the anterior wall of the vena cava, gently penetrating through the small bridge of tissue toward the junction of the medial hepatic vein and the left lateral hepatic vein. From above, a blunt, curved clamp is gently passed into the bifurcation of the median and left lateral hepatic vein, until the clamp is palpated on the posterior surface of the liver. A sling placed around the left hepatic vein facilitates identification of the correct line of dissection later in the procedure.

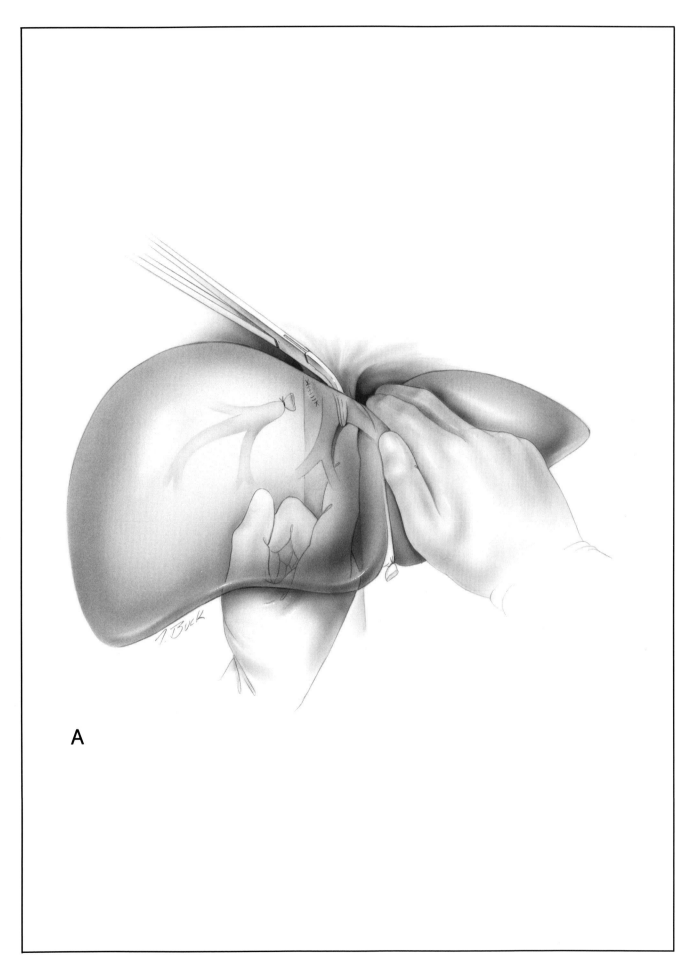

A

B The procedure starts as for a standard right hepatectomy, with complete preparation of the hilum. A cholecystectomy is performed after full identification of the structures in Calot's triangle. The right hepatic duct is identified and severed, its proximal end simply suture-ligated at the surface of the liver and the distal edge secured by a running monofilament 5-0 suture, avoiding any narrowing of the left duct. The right hepatic artery is dissected free and the bifurcation to the left and right hepatic arteries exposed. Following clear identification of the arterial supply to the left lobe, the right hepatic artery is divided and doubly ligated. Beneath the hepatic artery, the right branch of the portal vein is usually identified directly at the bifurcation of the portal vein. The vessel is divided between curved vascular clamps and the proximal orifice is oversewn by running 5-0 monofilament sutures. Following the oversewing of the distal stump at the liver surface, the parenchyma should now be demarcated. The resection continues at the posterior surface of the liver.

C With a tourniquet encircling the hepatoduodenal ligament and the infrahepatic vena cava, the right lobe is gently rolled over toward the left side and the accessory hepatic veins, draining directly into the inferior vena cava, are exposed. Each hepatic vein branch is carefully identified and a small, curved vascular clamp placed at its caval end for safety. The delicate veins are suture-ligated extremely carefully with 4-0 or 5-0 monofilament suture. This maneuver gradually allows exposure of the posterior surface of the liver and the anterior surface of the cava, so that the right hepatic vein can be identified. To perform an extended right hepatectomy, all hepatic veins entering the entire anterior surface of the vena cava must be disconnected from the liver parenchyma.

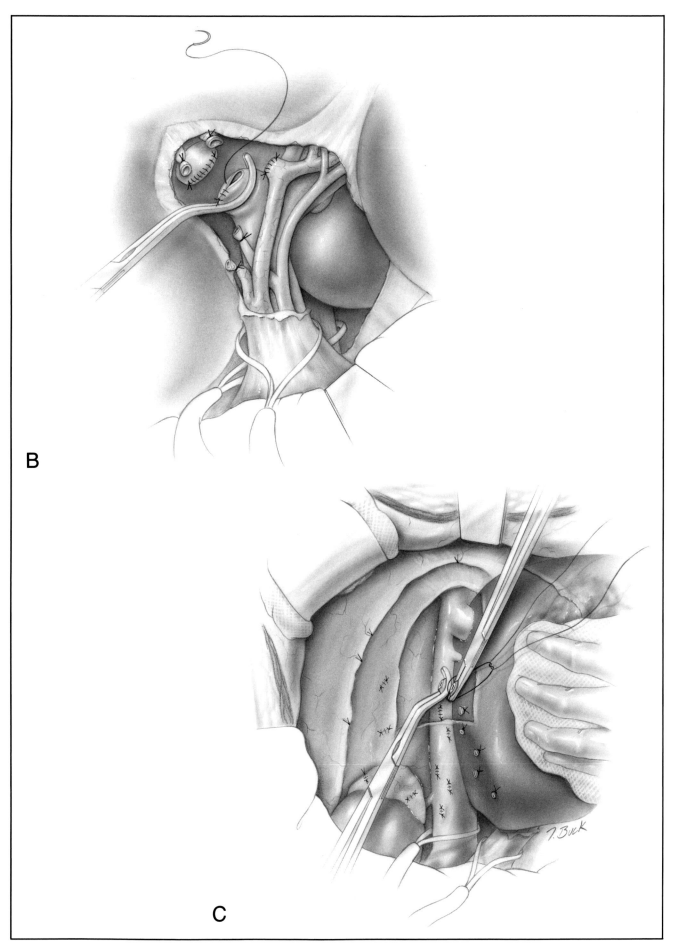

B

C

Under full visualization, the right hepatic vein is encircled by gently passing a curved vascular clamp between the middle and right hepatic veins. A second clamp is placed high against the liver and the vessel divided. Both ends are oversewn with 4-0 monofilament suture. At this point, the right portion of the vena cava is completely exposed and freed, but the left lobe still maintains its vascular supply and hepatic venous outflow.

The resection returns to the hilar dissection by continuing to mobilize the portal vein for identification of the branch to the median left segment. Usually this is the first branch coming off distal to the bifurcation of the right and left portal vein. Following its identification, the branch is clamped proximally and distally and divided. At the proximal end, a running suture with 5-0 monofilament suture is performed. Distally, a simple suture-ligation prevents sanguinous backflow.

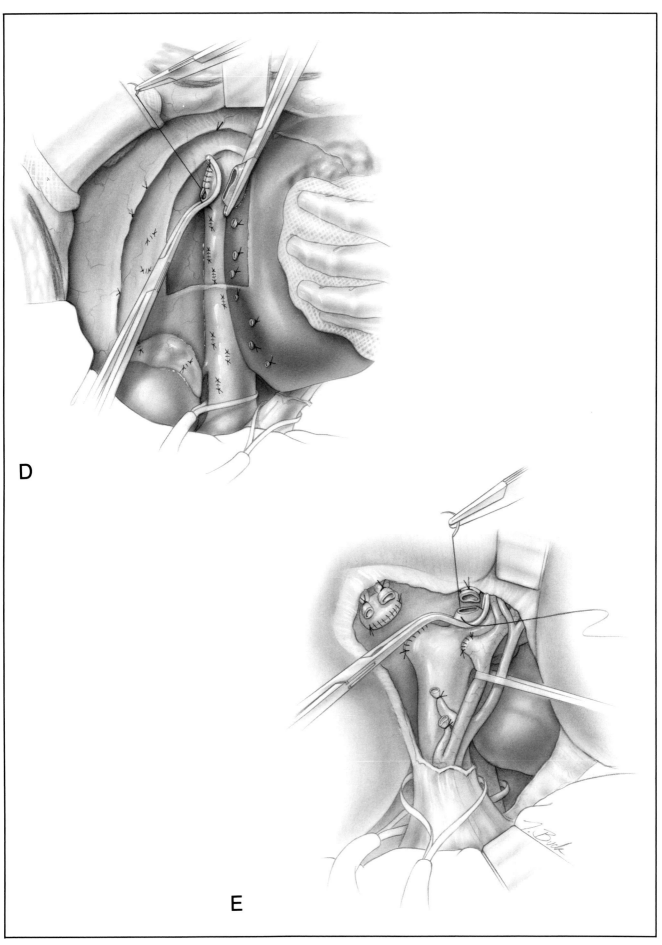

D

E

F
G

With the portal venous branch disconnected, the left hepatic duct and the left hepatic artery need to be followed into the lateral margin of the round ligament. At this location a peritoneal layer can be dissected sharply, revealing the arterial branch supplying the median left segment beneath. The artery to the median left segment should be clearly identified. Only if there is a clear, palpable pulse in the artery supplying the remaining left lateral segment should the first branches be ligated. If there is any doubt about the exact anatomy and arterial supply, the artery should remain untouched. The same is true for the exploration of the left hepatic duct. Usually a separate bile duct collects the bile from the median left segment to enter into the left hepatic duct. Once the artery is disconnected, the bile duct lies just next to it and can be identified with gentle, blunt dissection into the liver parenchyma. In most cases, a small duct can be identified arising from the median segment and should be disconnected sharply, leaving enough margin of tissue to suture-ligate the orifice entering into the left hepatic duct without causing stenosis. At this point, most of the median left hepatic segment should be devascularized, although some blood supply may be maintained from the left lateral artery through collaterals in the round ligament.

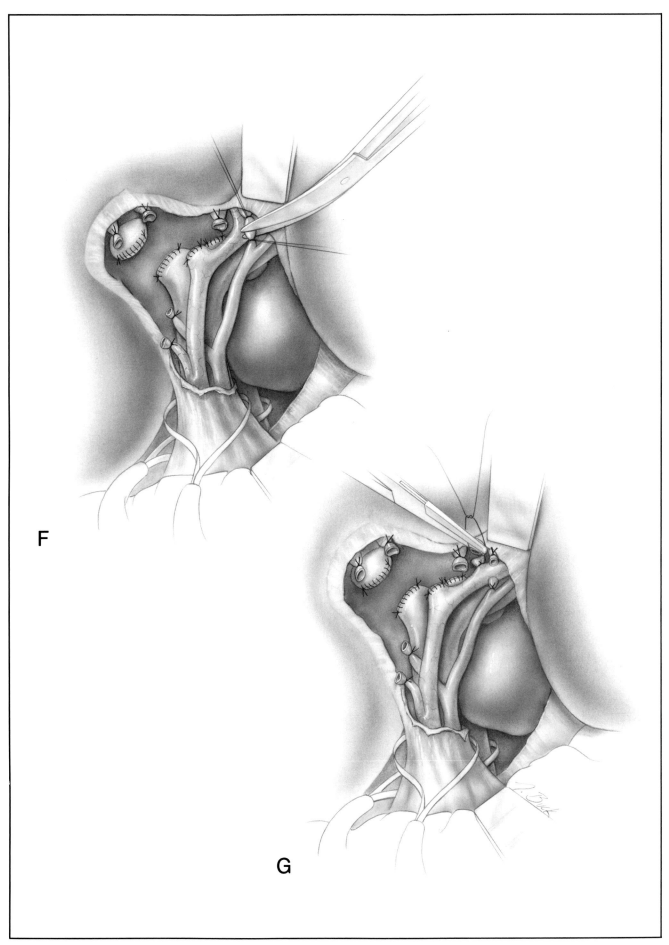

F

G

H The right and left lobes, being still attached to each other, are lifted more ventrally so that the posterior surface becomes exposed. Slight traction exerted in the hilum from the right and posterior side exposes the left median hepatic vein. It can be safely clamped with small, curved vascular clamps, severed and oversewn with running 5-0 monofilament suture.

I Suturing the orifice of the left median hepatic vein avoids unnecessary traction on the left lateral vein. However, on no account should this remaining single vein be stenosed, and care must be taken to avoid any traumatic laceration of this thin and nonelastic vessel.

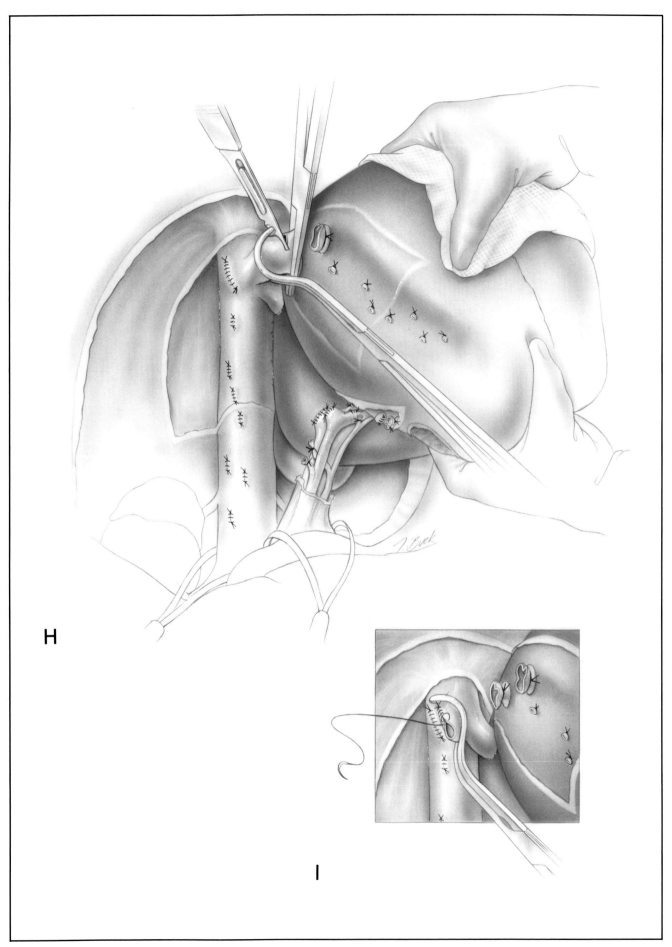

H

I

J After surgical dissection of the hilum and full exposure of the vena cava and posterior surface of the liver, the entire liver is placed back into its anatomic position following the disconnection of the hepatic veins. Note that only a small portion of the falciform ligament is incised, and the entire portion of the left triangular ligament remains in place. The blood supply through the falciform ligament can be a substantial nutritional factor to the liver, particularly in maintaining its arterial blood supply through the capsules and collaterals. The entire right lobe and the median left segment are thus completely devascularized, apart from a small portion of the median left segment adjacent to the lateral segments.

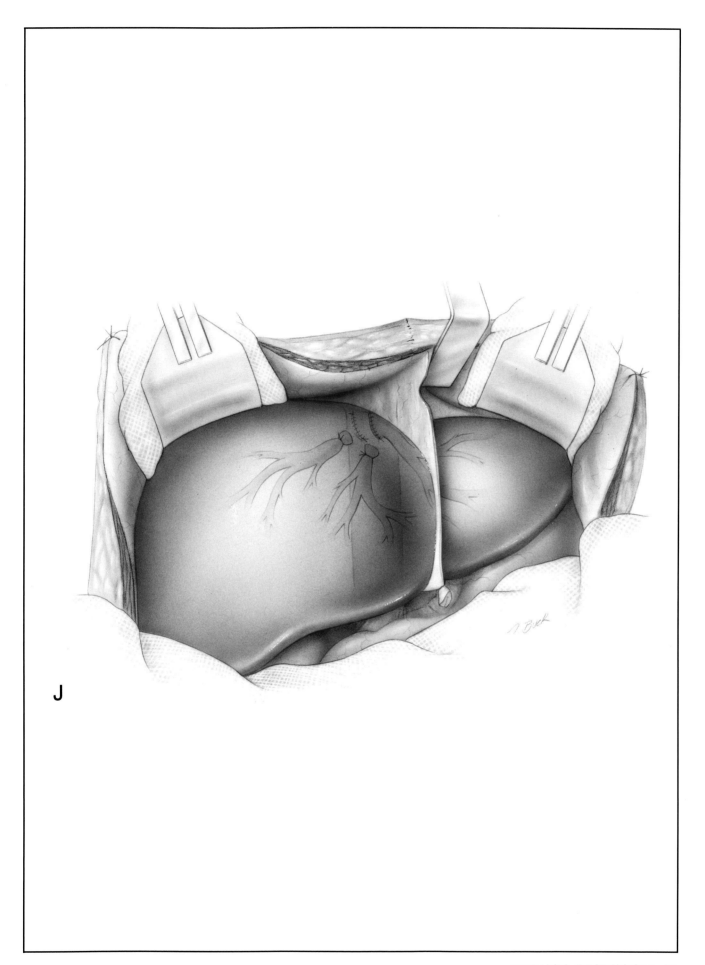

J

Without interruption of the blood flow to the left lateral segments, the parenchymal dissection is carried out adjacent to the falciform ligament. With the right hand, the surgeon puts his index finger underneath the posterior surface of the liver, while the thumb gently compresses the cut edge of the parenchyma to the right lateral side. The left hand performs the electrocautery. The assistant places his index finger parallel to the surgeon's index finger, gently controlling the hilar structures and the anterior parenchyma medial to the falciform ligament.

With manual compression by the assistant ("sandwich technique"), the parenchymal dissection proceeds along the posterior surface of the liver, parallel to both the round and falciform ligaments. The few vessels crossing this plane mainly arise from the round ligament and can be identified and ligated individually. Bleeding is controlled by suture placement directly through the cut liver edge. The tissue of the right lobe is gently pulled toward the right side. This maneuver further clarifies the vascular and biliary anatomy, and the branches to the lateral segments can be clearly visualized if identification at an earlier stage has proved difficult. At this point, they can be severed close to the cut edge of the right lobe in order not to compromise the circulation to the remaining left lateral segment. Under this visualization, they can be easily controlled and suture-ligated.

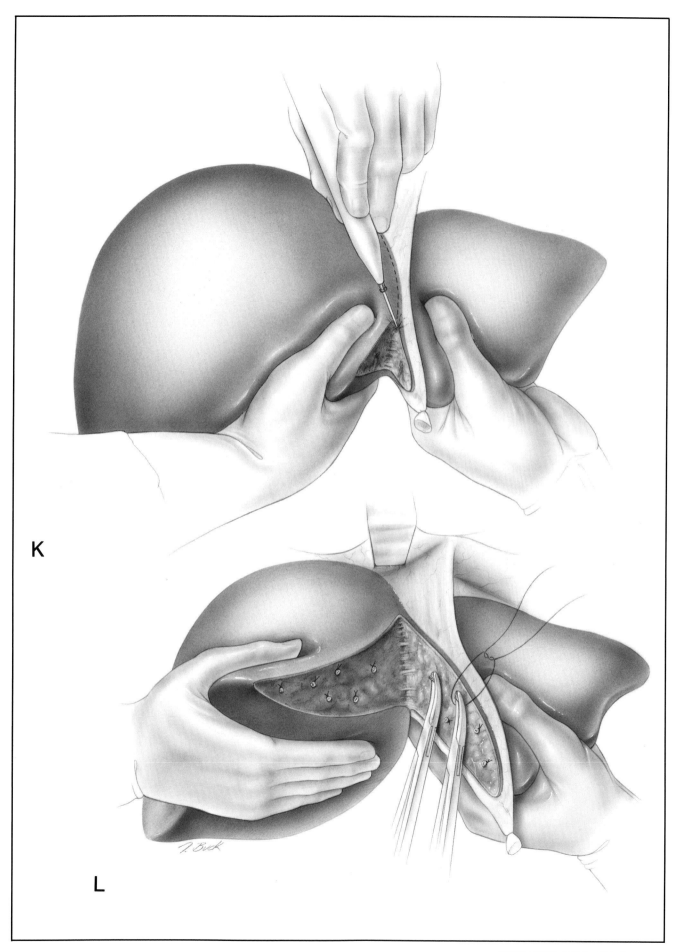

K

L

After the parenchymal dissection is performed, a relatively small area of dissected tissue lateral to the falciform ligament is exposed. Bleeding points or minor biliary leaks can be easily identified and controlled by suture-ligation. The risks of complications from this cut surface are much lower compared to those following a standard left or right hepatectomy. Since the falciform ligament and the left triangular ligament are left in place, twisting or torsion of the remaining left hepatic vein becomes almost impossible. The extremely large cavity of the right subdiaphragmatic fossa can be reduced in size by the placement of omental flaps and hepatic colonic flexure following full mobilization. Diaphragmatic plication is usually not indicated, but percutaneous drainage through an "easy-flow" drain is strongly recommended.

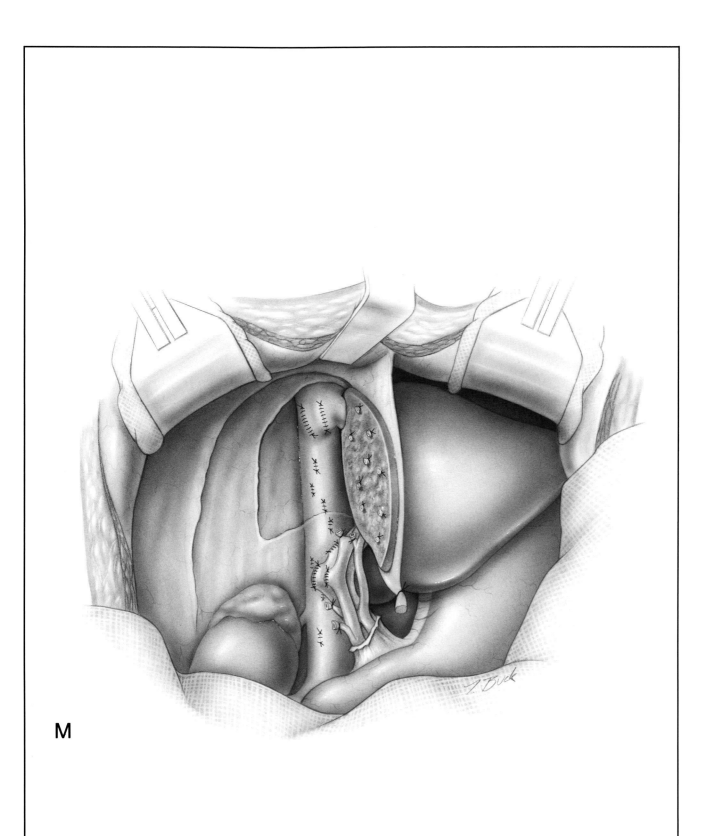

M

8 | Extended Right Hepatectomy Including Reconstruction of the Inferior Vena Cava

Extended right hepatectomies are rarely indicated for large primary hepatocellular tumors. However, tumors with a relatively good prognosis include the fibrolamellar-type of carcinoma and hepatoblastomas in young children. Aggressive surgery can be curative and may be necessary to achieve several years of palliation and excellent quality of life. Extensive preoperative evaluation should clarify whether the major veins, including the vena cava, are involved in the tumor process. Compression involvement of the inferior vena cava does not exclude hepatic resection, provided the tumor can be freed from the retroperitoneum and has not invaded the hilar structures. Again, jaundice and involvement of the hepatic artery are contraindications to resection.

When a tumor is located in the central portion of the right lobe with potential involvement of the inferior vena cava, resectability is determined by two factors: patency of the left portal vein and left hepatic artery, and lack of invasion of the retroperitoneum. To explore the latter, the right triangular ligament is dissected and the right lobe of the liver fully mobilized. The adrenal veins are exposed and suture-ligated and the entire retroperitoneum must be visualized. Only then can a decision be made as to whether the tumor has invaded the retroperitoneum and whether the hepatic venous outflow is free from involvement.

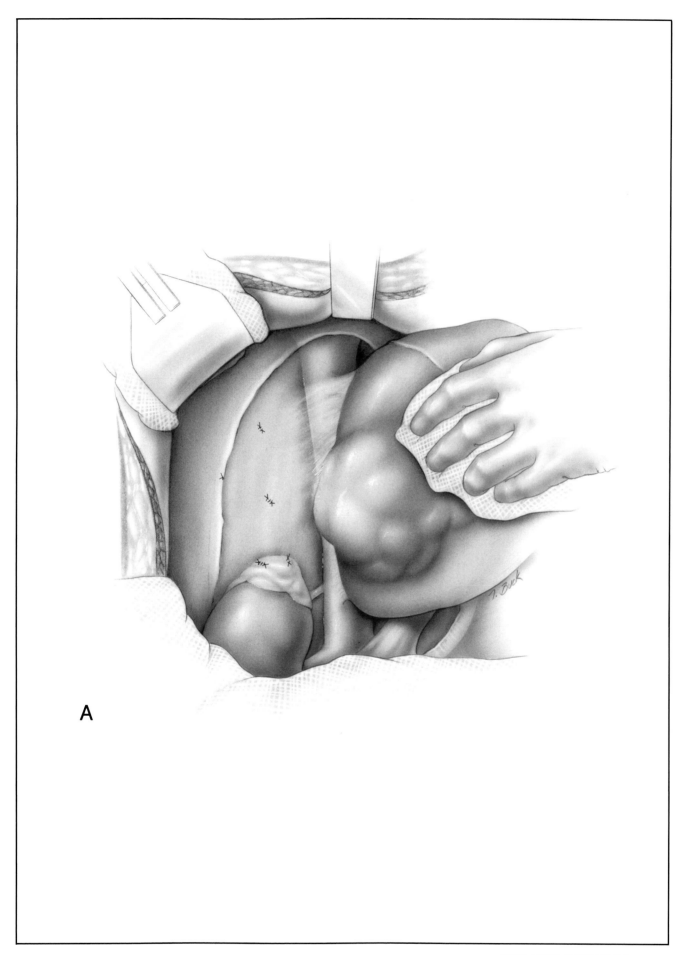

A

For this extended procedure it becomes necessary to control bleeding from the vena cava above and below the liver. To control the suprahepatic vena cava, the falciform ligament is dissected down to the anterior portion of the vena cava. With a combination of digital manipulation and gentle, blunt dissection, the vena cava is surrounded above the entrance of the right and left hepatic vein. Control is achieved either by a tourniquet or, preferably, by a specially designed vascular/diaphragmatic clamp, which prevents slipping of the vena cava once the vessel has been occluded within the extension of the diaphragm.

Control of the vena cava below the liver can be obtained with a straight vascular clamp and by placing a tourniquet around the hepatoduodenal ligament. A vascular clamp is preferred over occlusion by tourniquet, since the former facilitates venous reconstruction.

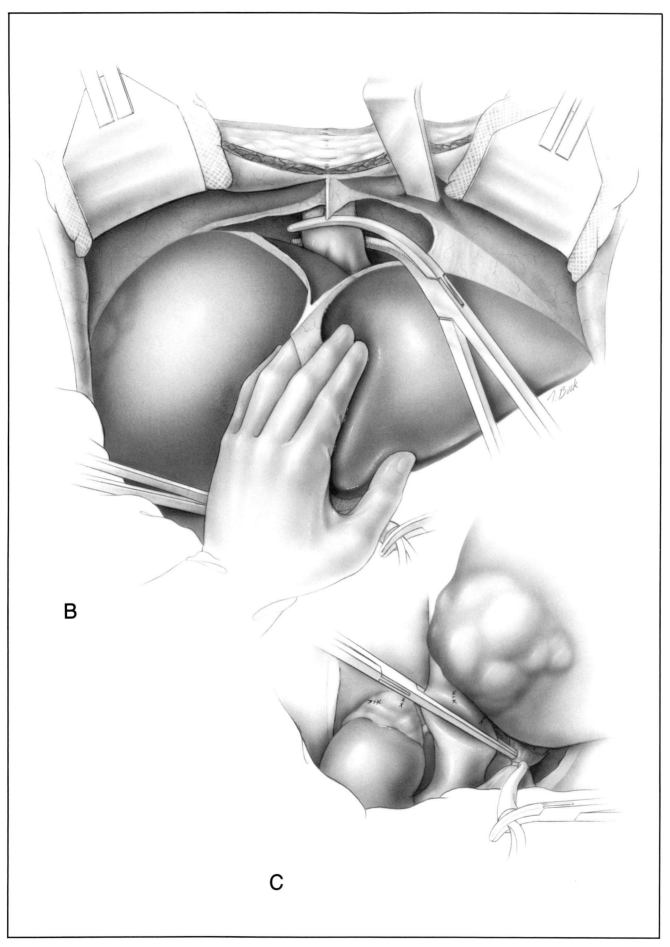

B

C

After resectability has been confirmed and control of the vena cava is obtained above and below the liver, the dissection at the hilum can proceed in the usual fashion. The right hepatic duct is suture-ligated first, followed by the right branch of the portal vein. The right hepatic artery is identified and the left hepatic artery preserved. With gentle dissection of the left branch of the portal vein, the first branch supplying the left median segment is identified and suture-ligated. Separate arterial and biliary branches are identified and similarly suture-ligated.

The caudate lobe is mobilized and freed by dissecting through the lesser omentum. It is essential that the left lateral hepatic vein and the median hepatic vein are individually identified before dissection of the parenchyma starts. Dependent on the extension of the tumor within the liver, the rest of the procedure is done under total vascular exclusion. The tourniquet around the hepatoduodenal ligament is tightened, and the inferior vena cava is cross-clamped above the renal veins and directly below the diaphragm.

Although some surgeons perform in situ cooling of the whole liver at this juncture, we have found this unnecessary, since this procedure rarely takes more than 45 minutes. Warm ischemia of this duration rarely produces clinical problems. Dissection of the parenchyma is performed expeditiously, using a combination of electrocautery and mosquito clamp and fracture techniques. With slight traction of the occluded hilar structure, the posterior surface of the liver is reached from sagittal penetration into the parenchyma.

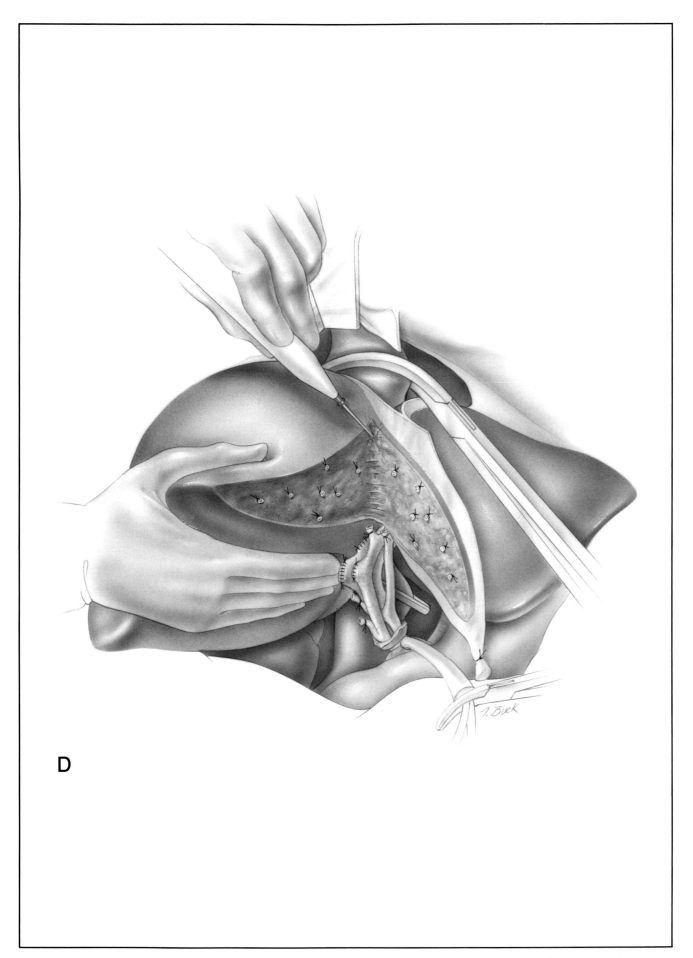

D

E Following the complete dissection of the parenchyma, the tumor involving the inferior vena cava becomes evident. Lifting the right lobe out of the hepatic fossa allows transection of the cava, and the upper margin leaves enough cava so that the left hepatic vein remains undisturbed. The right hepatic vein is suture-ligated to preserve some length of the infradiaphragmatic vena cava, and to prevent outflow obstruction for the remaining left lateral hepatic vein.

F To remove the tumor-cava complex, clamps (both above and below the liver) are positioned, while the right lobe of the liver containing the tumor and the segment of the inferior vena cava involved are removed. The hepatoduodenal ligament is occluded by the tourniquet and gently pulled over to the left side. The bleeding from the lumbar veins must be secured together with hemorrhage from the retroperitoneum. At this point, a decision can be made as to whether in situ cooling should be implemented. If the time necessary to perform the procedure and secure adequate hemostasis is greater than 45 minutes, a cannula should be placed in the left portal vein, via the right portal vein stump, and ice-cold perfusate instilled. A small hole is made in the right hepatic stump to allow drainage of the perfusate if the clamp is above the hepatic venous complex. If the clamp is below the left hepatic vein, then the perfusate simply flows into the cava.

Although we do not generally advocate in situ cooling or the application of extracorporeal portal vein decompression using a veno-venous bypass system, we have used this procedure in several cases where the reconstruction time was expected to be longer than 1 hour. This option should be reserved for exceptional cases, and should only be used by surgeons experienced in its use (i.e., liver transplant surgeons).

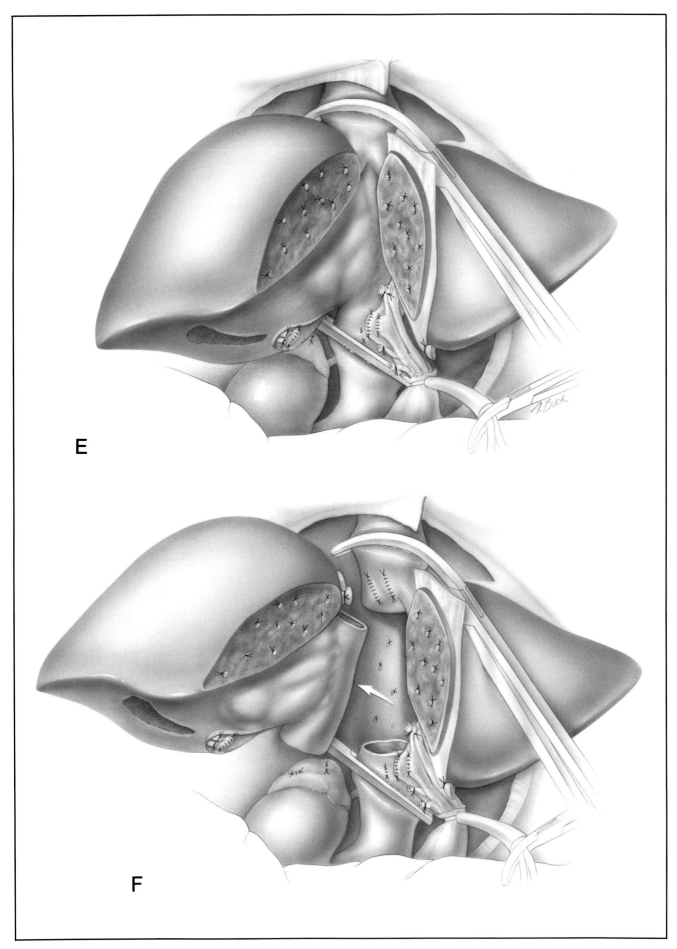

E

F

G Reconstruction of the inferior vena cava is performed using a large diameter Dacron or Gore-Tex prosthesis (e.g., 2.5 cm). Total cross-clamping and occlusion of the hepatoduodenal ligament requires rapid reconstruction of the proximal end of the inferior vena cava, since the first goal is to restore blood circulation through the left lateral segment and allow for free hepatic venous outflow. The upper margin is anastomosed using continuous 3-0 monofilament suture. If the clamp has been placed above the left hepatic vein, it should be exchanged for another placed below it, to allow drainage of the left lateral lobe.

H Once the upper anastomosis has been performed, the cross-clamping can be released and the clamp replaced caudal to the entry of the left lateral hepatic vein. The clamp can even be placed below the anastomosis while the lower anastomosis is sutured circumferentially. A 4-0 monofilament suture is used, with an atraumatic needle. Before the suture of the lower anastomosis is completed, air must be evacuated from the Dacron prosthesis by allowing a backflow of blood through the graft. The clamps are finally released. Hemorrhaging and bile leakage are carefully controlled from the cut surface and from all suture-ligated orifices. "Easy-flow" drains are placed, and an omentum flap is positioned on top and around the vascular prosthesis.

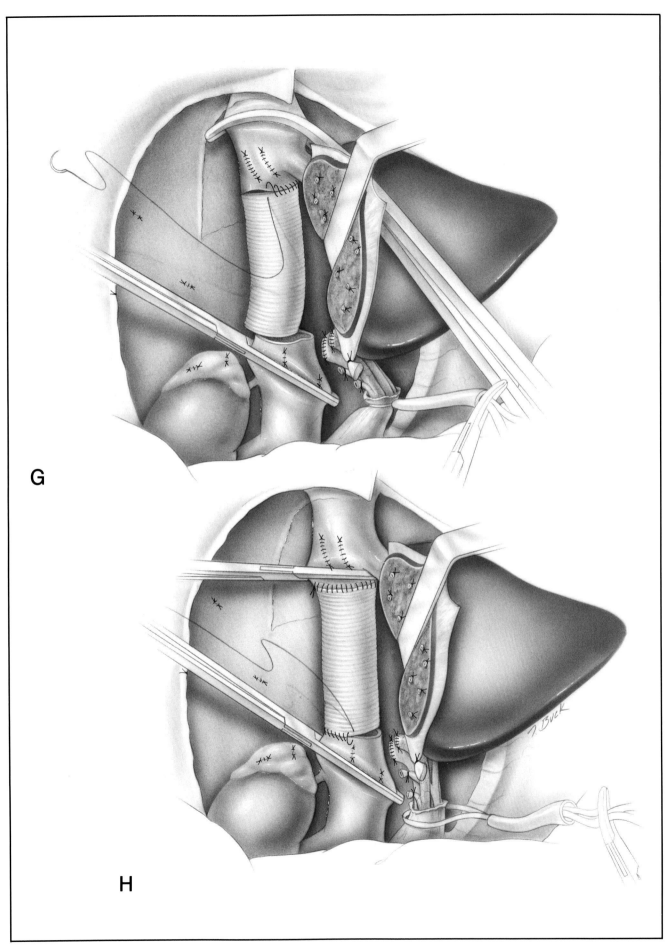

G

H

9 | Left Lateral (Nonanatomic) Hepatectomy

The left lateral hepatectomy is one of the most commonly performed nonanatomic hepatic resections for lesions confined to the left lateral segment. Solitary metastases are easily removed by this procedure. Although all patients undergoing hepatic resection should have a standard work-up, a nonanatomic resection of the left lobe does not specifically require angiography. However, one should be aware that, in more than 15 percent of these cases, unsuspected lesions in the right and median left lobe of the liver can be present and may be identified by selective angiography. For this reason, we would still recommend it.

Lesions are amenable to left lateral segmentectomy when they are confined exclusively to the left lateral segment and are far enough away from the falciform ligament to leave a tumor-free margin of at least 1 cm. The risk of this procedure is relatively small, even in the presence of liver cirrhosis.

A formal Mercedes incision is not mandatory for this type of procedure; a midline incision will suffice. This incision can always be extended under the right costal margin if a more extended resection ensues. This approach avoids the unnecessary large transverse incision so often used, and is particularly beneficial if disseminated disease precludes hepatic resection.

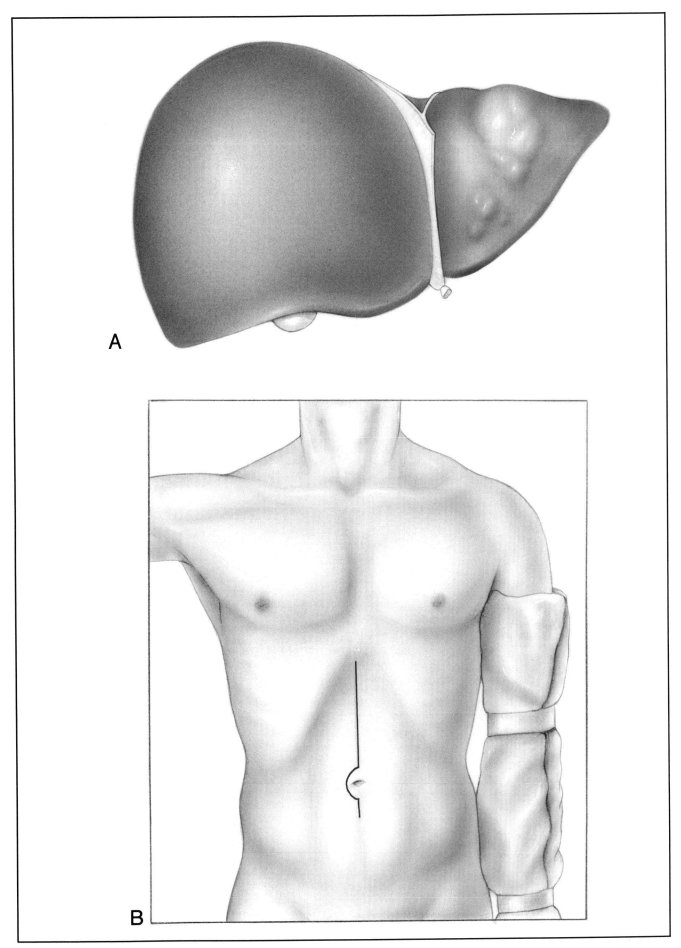

A

B

C
D

Retractors are placed to allow full exposure of the left liver, with access to the falciform ligament and left triangular ligament. Following careful manual exploration and, whenever possible, intraoperative ultrasound, the falciform ligament is dissected close to the diaphragm until the left hepatic vein is exposed. The dissection proceeds on the left side with electrocautery of the left triangular ligament.

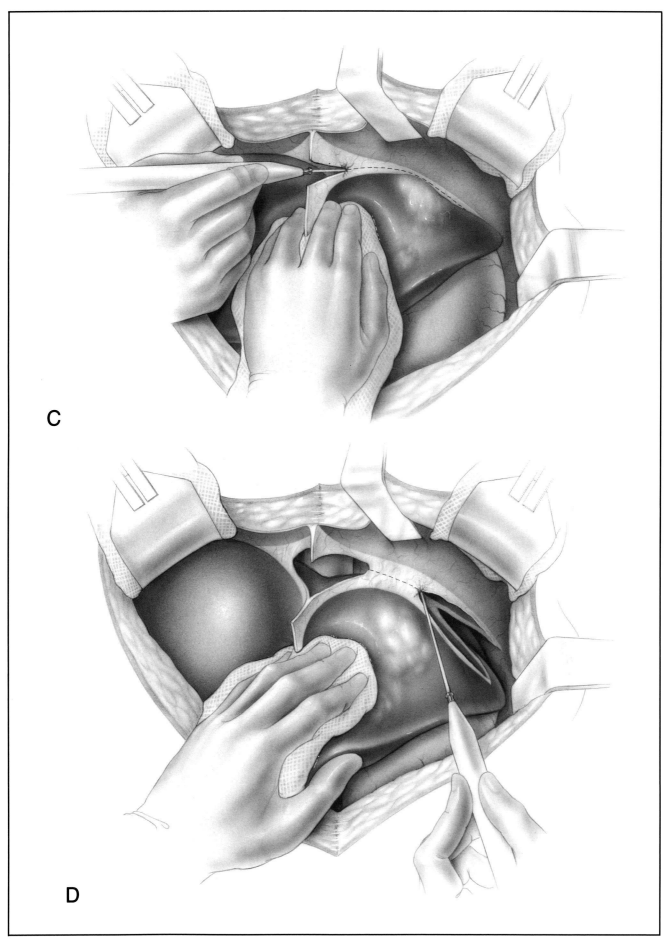

C

D

The posterior surface of the left lateral segment is exposed by gentle retraction, and the lesser omentum and the lesser curvature of the stomach are exposed. The lesser omentum is dissected close to the liver without disturbing the gastric arcades. In the event of a left hepatic artery arising from the left gastric artery, it can be dissected and carefully suture-ligated on both sides. The dissection proceeds near the hilum and follows the extension of the round ligament posteriorly. It continues caudally until the left lateral hepatic vein can be identified as it enters the inferior vena cava. Frequently, a large diaphragmatic vein drains into the left lateral hepatic vein, as it enters the vena cava. This confluence can be left undisturbed as the upper margin of dissection.

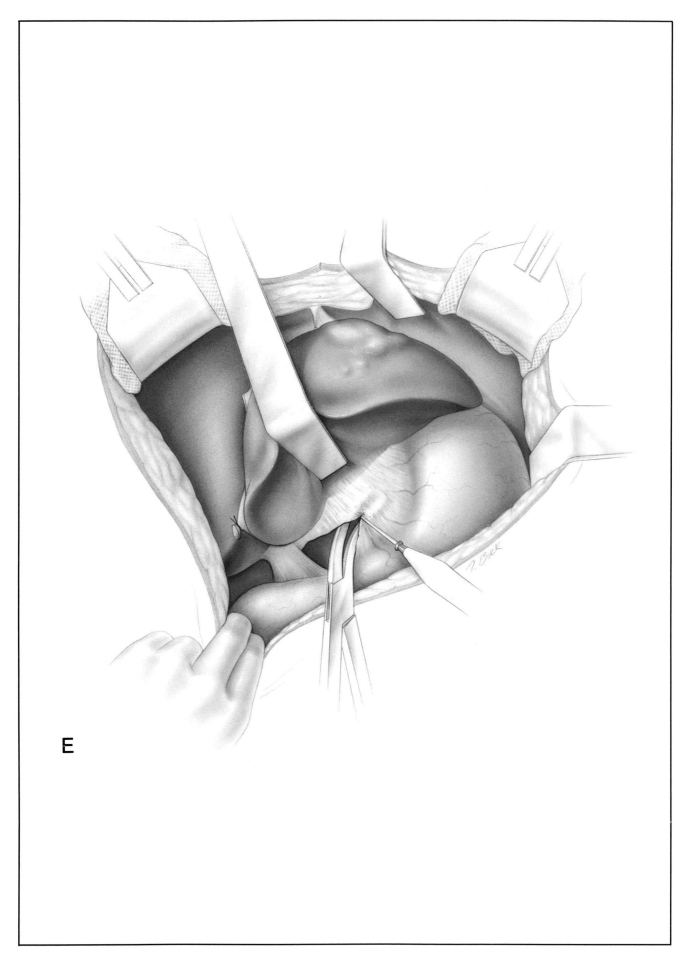

E

F With the posterior surface of the left lateral segment clearly dissected and the landmarks of the hilum and the left lateral hepatic vein identified, the relatively small bridge of hepatic parenchyma connecting the left lateral segment with the median segment can be approached for parenchymal dissection. The assistant secures the left median segment between his index finger and thumb, compressing it like a sandwich. This allows the surgeon to place mattress sutures medially to the falciform ligament through the depth of the whole left lateral segment. For this procedure, 2-0 chromic catgut or 2-0 monofilament suture on atraumatic needles can be used. It is essential that the sutures be placed evenly, no more than 0-5 cm apart. While the surgeon ties each suture, the assistant exerts slight compression with his index finger and thumb to allow the placement of the knot. In this way, with careful coordination between surgeon and assistant, tearing of the liver parenchyma is rare. The use of absorbable pledgets can be avoided in most cases. However, whenever tighter compression is needed, the stitches can be placed through the round ligament at the posterior surface of the lobe and the residual falciform ligament on the anterior surface.

G Mattress sutures are placed through the liver parenchyma. It is important to note that the mattress sutures form a line of compression, and are placed sequentially from the round ligament to the posterior part of the lobe.

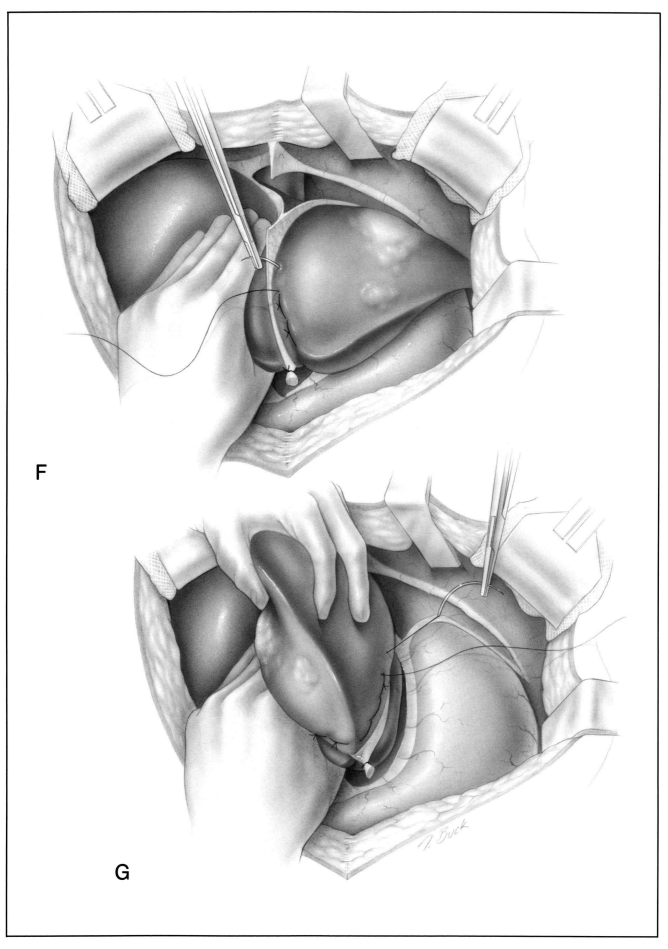

F

G

H The dissection of the parenchyma starts with electrocautery medial to the falciform ligament and the line of mattress sutures. At this point, the assistant can gently pull on the left lateral segment to allow access to the cut surface. Individual clamps may have to be placed on vascular or biliary structures that are greater than 1 mm. After the parenchymal transection, additional individual suture-ligations may have to secure bleeding points or small biliary leaks not completely controlled by the mattress sutures.

I When the dissection and removal of the left lateral segment is completed, careful attention must be paid to exclude residual arterial or venous bleeding or bile leakage. Bile leakage from the cut surface is the most common postoperative complication, with an incidence of 5 to 10 percent. Additional mattress sutures should include a piece of the falciform ligament or round ligament from the posterior surface. Minor oozing can be troublesome, but may be controlled by utilizing either infrared light coagulation or argon beam coagulation, or even with fibrin glue. Compression with a warm abdominal pack is both useful and simple. Principally, whenever there is no bleeding, no additional procedures are necessary. Should there be significant bleeding, it should be controlled surgically with sutures. The methods described above will not control *persistent* hemorrhage. After completion of the procedure, the cut surface should be drained.

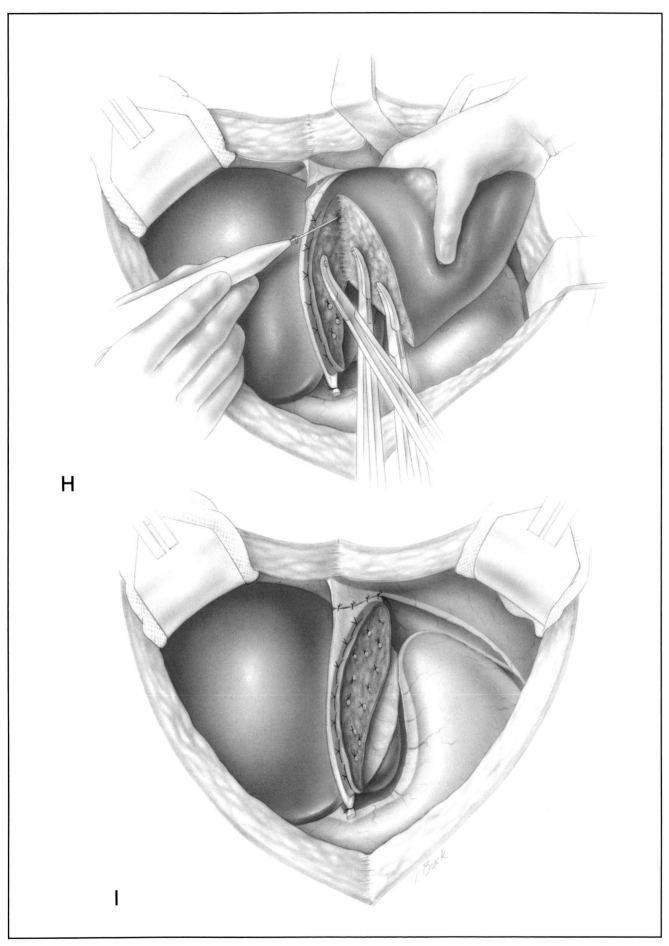

H

I

10 | Median Hepatectomy (Removal of Segment 4)

Centrally located tumors may be resectable by removing only the median left segment. This type of tumor would include solitary metastatic disease in the area, as well as tumors lying at or near the confluence of the bile ducts. It should be remembered that the median left lobe functions as an independent lobe, with its own portal and vascular supply and its own biliary drainage. The duct from this segment joins the left lateral duct to form the main left hepatic duct at the base of the round ligament. It is at this junction, for example, that, in cases of obstruction in the hilum of the liver, the dilated bile duct in the left lateral lobe can be drained (segment 3 bypass operation), which has the advantage of also draining the median left lobe.

Confining the resection to removing only the median left segment preserves the functional parenchyma of the right or left lobe, while still maintaining adequate tumor-free margins. Anatomically, a full left lobectomy would be needed to eliminate a lesion in the left median segment, but this incorporates the unnecessary removal of 20 percent of functional liver parenchyma.

A In the case of a centrally located tumor, the line of resection is represented by the interrupted line running along the falciform ligament and along the plane between the right and left lobes, from the bed of the gallbladder to the cava.

B After performing a cholecystectomy, the hepatoduodenal ligament is dissected by opening the covering peritoneal layers. Once the cystic duct and the cystic artery are ligated, the incision continues to the left to identify the confluence of the bile duct and the bifurcation of the hepatic artery.

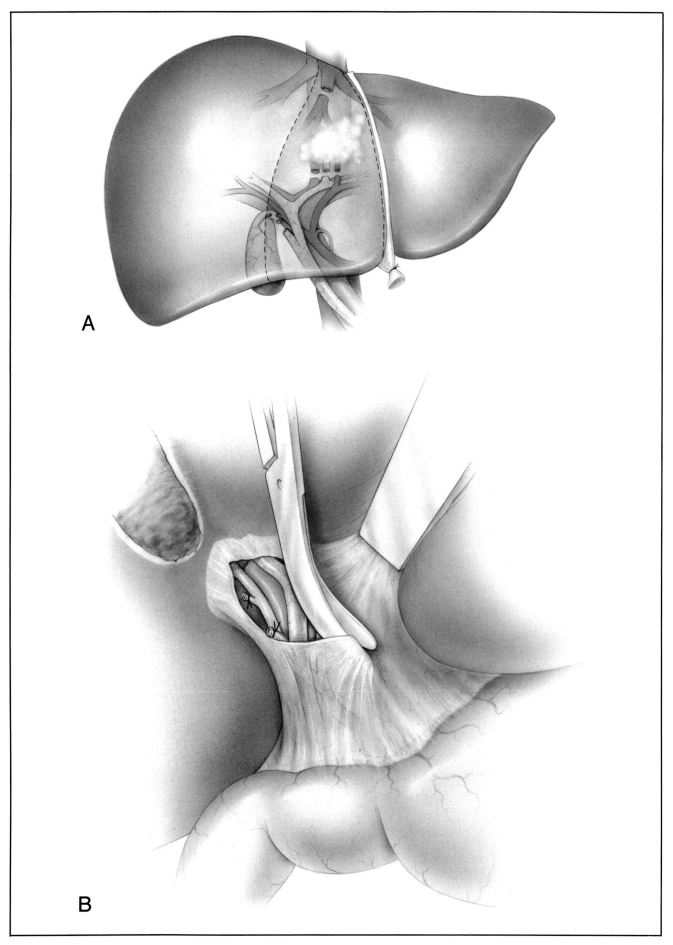

A

B

C A standard cholecystectomy is performed first. Calot's triangle is exposed, and a tourniquet is placed loosely around the hepatoduodenal ligament. The cava should also be dissected and slung with a tourniquet, but not occluded. The hepatic artery is identified and traced to its bifurcation. The dissection continues along the left hepatic artery to identify the small branch that feeds the median left segment. Usually, this artery branches off before the left hepatic artery dives into the base of the round ligament to enter the parenchyma. The left hepatic bile duct is sometimes a useful landmark, since this artery tends to cross over the left hepatic bile duct at the margin of the parenchyma. At this point, the artery to the median segment can usually be suture-ligated and divided. The main trunk of the left hepatic artery must not be damaged or occluded. Care should also be taken not to traumatize the adjacent left hepatic duct, which continues to run parallel to the artery at the base of the round ligament. The bile duct branch draining the left median segment usually lies just beneath the artery, and can be found by simply lifting the artery gently with a rubber vessel loop.

D Proceeding into the hilum of the liver, the confluence of the left and right hepatic bile ducts must be clearly identified. The left hepatic duct is followed along the left hepatic artery until a small duct is found arising from the median segment. This branch is usually half the size of the left hepatic duct, and requires formal suture-ligation to prevent bile leakage.

Following mobilization of the left hepatic bile duct, the bifurcation of the right and left portal vein branches can be easily identified. The first branch of the left portal vein, passing an anteriocranial direction, usually represents the portal vein branch feeding the left median segment. This branch needs to be identified, circled, and subsequently suture-ligated. In order not to compromise the blood flow to the remaining left lateral segment, a special clamp can be placed to occlude most of the lumen of the left portal venous branch, allowing suture-ligation with running 5-0 monofilament suture. After releasing the clamp, full blood flow to the left portal venous branch is restored. At this point, demarcation of the devascularized median left segment has usually occurred, although in many instances the anterior portion of the left median segment receives substantial blood supply through crossover branches from the round ligament, and may have no demarcation lines.

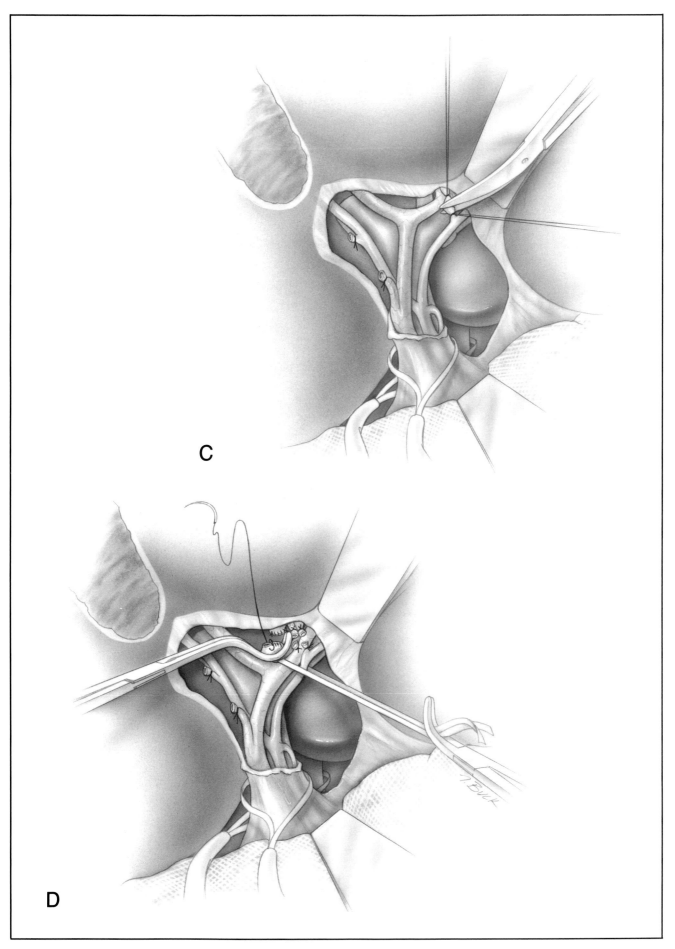

C

D

E In order to entirely devascularize the median left segment, the lateral portion of the round ligament must be dissected with step-by-step isolation of its vascular structures. The peritoneal layers surrounding the round ligament are sharply dissected, and portal venous branches (as well as small arterial branches) are identified, divided, and suture-ligated. By starting the dissection from the anterior surface and going to the base of the round ligament, a fissure between the left lateral segment and the left median segment can be created. By staying strictly on the lateral right side of the round ligament, no trauma to the remaining structures feeding the left lateral segment can occur.

A small bridge of liver parenchyma usually lies in front of the round ligament; it requires sharp dissection by electrocautery, and the suface should be oversewn with mattress sutures. Its dissection allows access to the bases of the round ligament and leads the way into the anatomic margin between the left lateral segment and the left median segment.

F The dissection of the parenchyma starts lateral to the round ligament and the falciform ligament. While the surgeon gently compresses the margin of the median left segment with his thumb from the posterior surface and his index finger around the anterior surface, the assistant performs the same technique on the medial side of the falciform and round ligaments with his index finger on top of the left lateral segment and his thumb on the posterior surface. Gentle traction is exerted on the round ligament to expose the base and the cut surface. Gradually, as the parenchyma is penetrated, medium- and large-sized structures are suture-ligated and divided. Blood loss is virtually zero at this stage. Of course, should bleeding occur, occlusion of the hepatoduodenal ligament could be performed, but the line of demarcation may diminish. It is therefore important to mark this line with electrocautery at the beginning of the procedure.

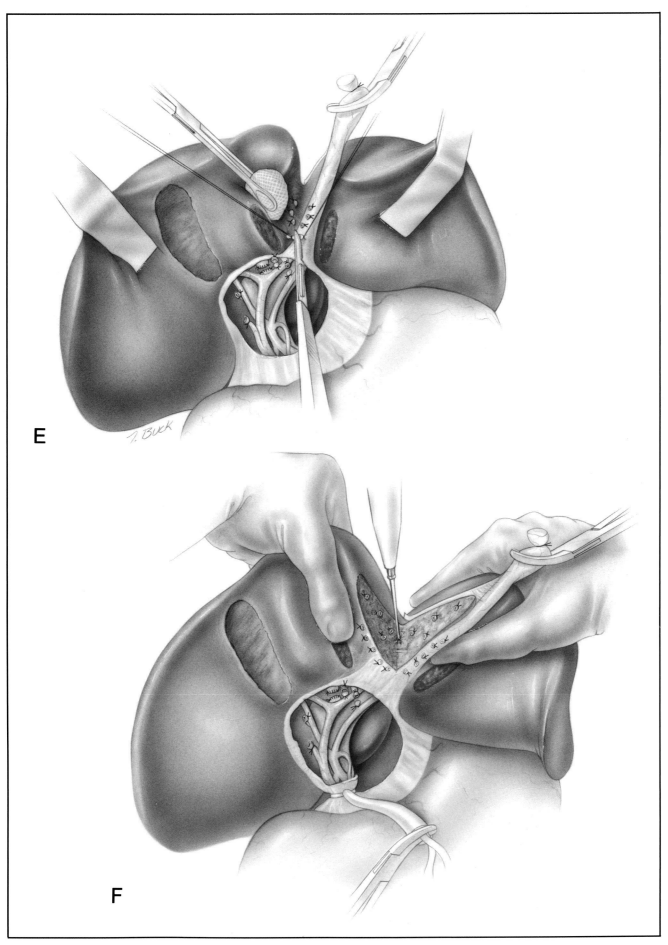

E

F

G

The dissection continues to the junction of the left median and left lateral hepatic veins. The left median vein needs to be carefully identified and then encircled and clamped with a special curved vascular clamp to allow its safe division. The hepatic vein is suture-ligated with continuous 5-0 monofilament suture on the caval side. If a Pringle maneuver (interruption of blood circulation through the hepatoduodenal ligament compression) was performed, it should now be released to re-identify the demarcation of the median left segment.

H

Along the anatomic line of demarcation, the separation of the median left segment from the right lobe starts by gentle compression of the parenchyma between the thumb and the index finger of the surgeon, placed around the right lobe. While the assistant holds the lateral margin of the left median segment with the same sandwich-compression technique, the parenchyma can be entered. The surgeon places mattress sutures along the margin of dissection. The sutures are tied with gentle compression and without laceration of the tissue. Large individual vessels require suture-ligation. To facilitate this procedure without unwarranted blood loss, the hepatoduodenal ligament can be occluded once again by the tourniquet. During the dissection maneuver, the anterior portion of the median left segment is flipped up anteriorly to visualize the vital structures of the hilum of the liver. Once clear identification of all the structures is obtained, the procedure of penetrating the parenchyma continues toward the area between the left and right hepatic veins. Since the median left hepatic vein has already been identified and divided, the line of dissection must remain close to the midline to avoid injury to the right hepatic vein as it enters the cava.

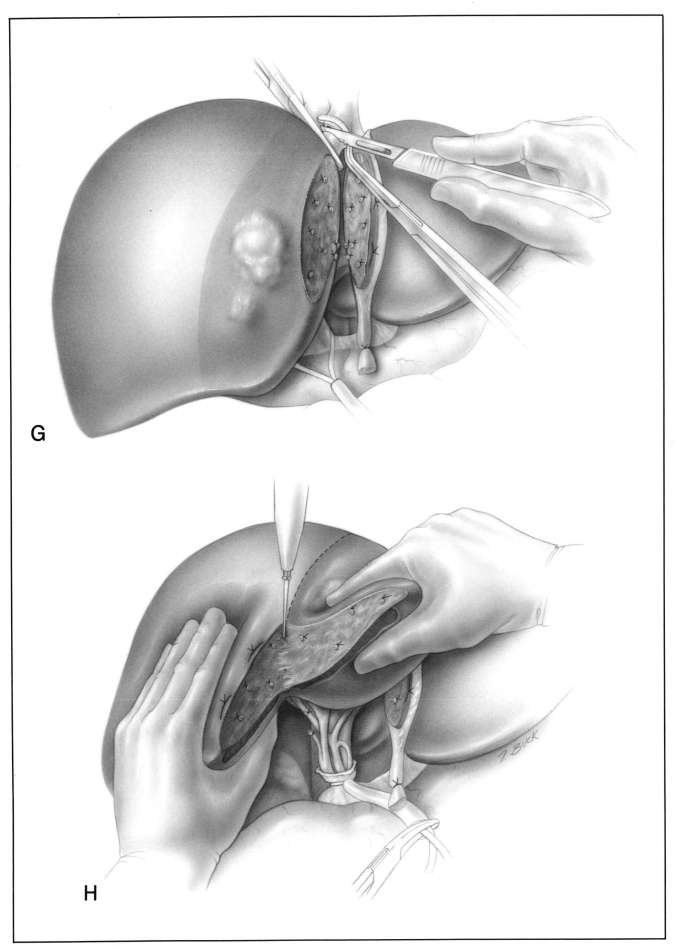

G

H

I   The parenchymal dissection to the left and right is completed, and the anterior surface of the inferior vena cava and the hilum of the liver are widely exposed. During the dissection of the posterior surface of the median left segment, careful attention must be paid in identifying hepatic veins that may be surrounded by margins of tissue. These hepatic veins should be carefully ligated without compromising the diameter of the cava. Should bleeding be encountered, the tourniquets on the cava and portal structures should be tightened. Careful, sharp dissection is less traumatic than blunt dissection in this situation, since these posterior veins are very thin and easily torn by traction.

This approach for a median left hepatectomy has been advocated for treatment of Klatskin tumors as well, since it allows the most extended exposure of the confluence of the left and right hepatic bile ducts, as well as of the bifurcation of the large nutrient vessels. For this procedure, of course, the dissection of the entire common hepatic duct is included in the elimination of the median left hepatic segment, leaving only the portal vein and branches of the right and left hepatic artery intact. However, for other types of hepatic resections, this procedure represents a major, difficult type of operation. Not only does it have to preserve all afferent vessels as well as two major hepatic veins, two large resection margins remain, which doubles the chances of a bile leak or postoperative bleeding.

The area between the left lateral segment and the right lobe may be covered with a flap of omentum if it can be mobilized into position. Approximating the two surfaces together offers no advantage, but this area should be adequately drained.

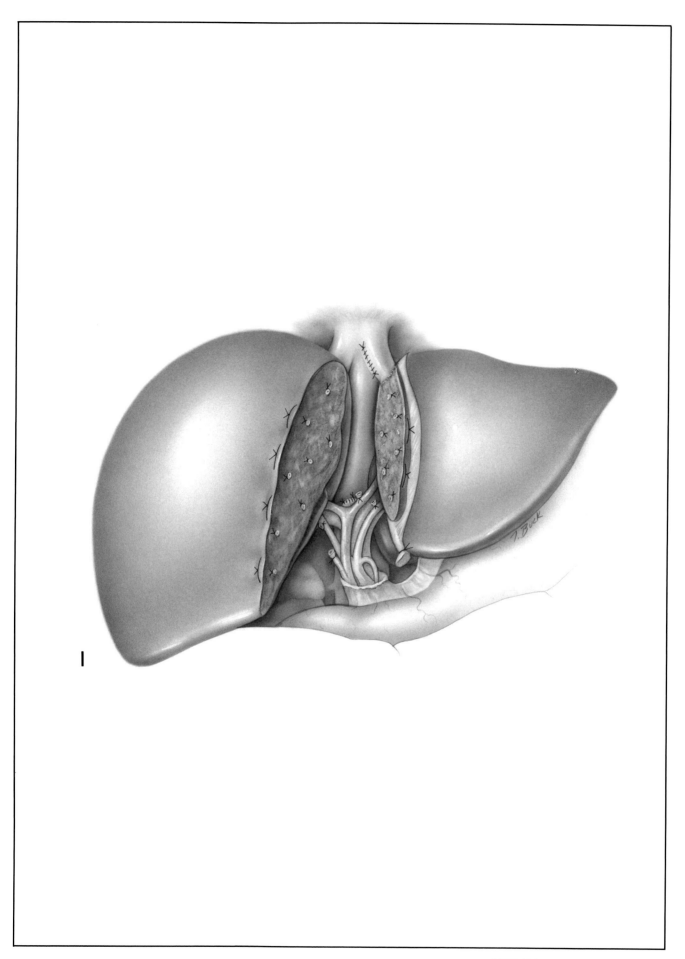

I

11 | Anatomic Left Lateral Hepatectomy

The anatomic left lateral hepatectomy with formal dissection of the hilum represents no distinct advantage over the conventional nonanatomic (wedge resection) of the left lateral segment for the majority of cases. However, the exposure of the individual structures supplying and draining the left lateral segment allows for a much more elegant approach, and is indicated when lesions in this area encroach on the round ligament, or when the depth of tissue through the line of resection is great. Mattress sutures in these situations may result in tissue necrosis and abscess formation. Furthermore, the dissection of the left lateral lobe forms the basis for performing segmental liver transplantation from living donors; this experience is essential and invaluable for an experienced transplant surgeon contemplating this procedure.

A | After complete division of the left triangular ligament, the hilum of the liver is widely exposed to include the course of the hepatic artery, the confluence of the left and right hepatic duct, and the underlying portal vein. The course of the common hepatic artery is followed and the existence of a left lateral hepatic artery, originating from the left gastric artery, must be identified if present.

B | The arterial supply to the left lateral segment can be dependent on an accessory hepatic artery arising from the left gastric artery, but the feeding branches to the left median segment usually arise from the left hepatic artery, originating from the common hepatic artery. For anatomic removal of the left lateral segment, the left lateral hepatic artery, regardless of its origin, requires dissection and ligation, and the artery feeding the median left hepatic segment should be preserved, its origin from the left hepatic arterial trunk clearly exposed and identified.

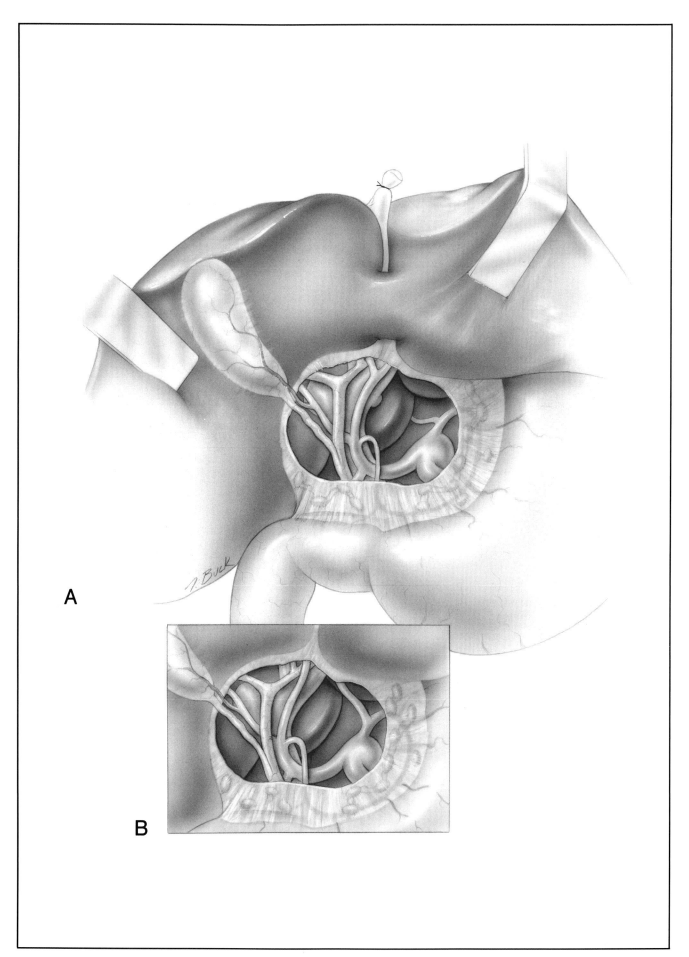

A

B

C The small bridge of tissue connecting the lower portion of the quadrate lobe with the posterior surface of the left lateral segment must be divided with electrocautery and bleeding controlled with mattress sutures. This maneuver facilitates exploration at the base of the round ligament.

D The liver is gently separated, allowing access to the round ligament; traction on the cut falciform ligament is helpful. The superficial peritoneal layer of the round ligament is dissected sharply to reveal the venous connections between it and the median left segment. These veins may bleed substantially and should be treated with caution. Ligation in continuity is advisable. We usually perform suture-ligation with a 5-0 monofilament suture on an atraumatic needle to prevent traumatizing of the surrounding tissue; this provides safe closure of even very small vessels. The dissection must free all the attachments of the round ligament until it is completely mobile.

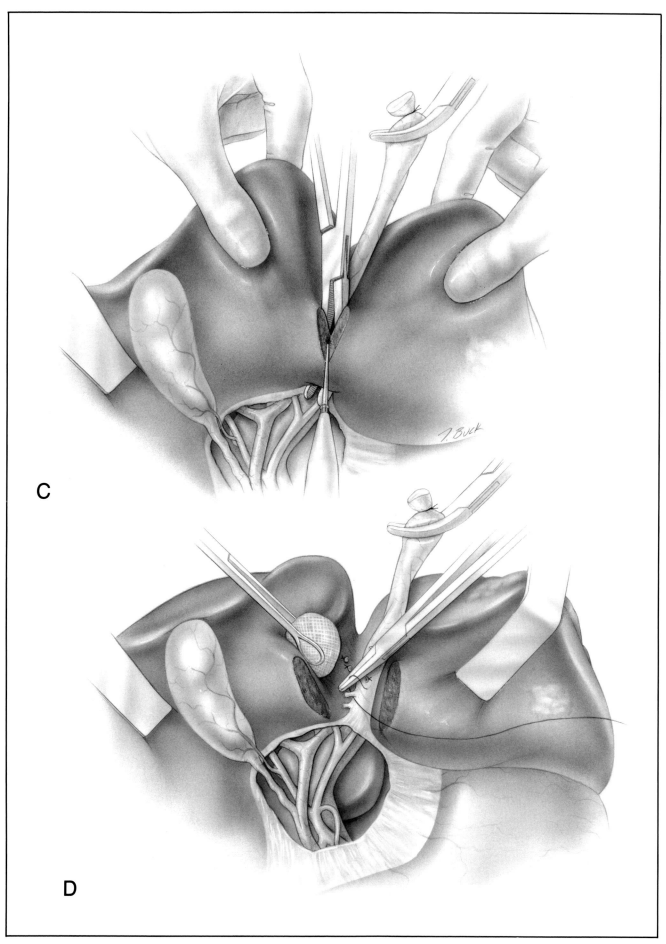

C

D

The left hepatic artery is traced into the left lateral segment. The branch(es) to the left median segment must be clearly identified and preserved. The branches to the left lateral segments can be divided between sutures. The portal vein can be exposed to gentle blunt dissection with a peanut swab, and is found directly beneath the artery. Finally, the bile ducts from the left lateral lobe and the left median lobe must be identified. Occasionally, the bile ducts arising from the lateral segments do not form a common trunk, and the bile duct from the median left segment joins the two separate ducts to form the main hepatic duct at the base of the round ligament. These ducts have to be clearly identified to preserve the duct from the middle segment. If identification proves difficult, dissection of the portal vein to the left lateral segment should be performed (see page 99). The ducts from the lateral lobe can be divided if visualized.

The portal vein to the left lobe can now be dissected and divided. Caution should be taken not to compromise the lumen of the right portal vein, but this is unlikely, since the division is distal to the branch supplying the caudate lobe and the left median segment. The portal vein is over-sewn with continuous monofilament, but the distal end need only be ligated.

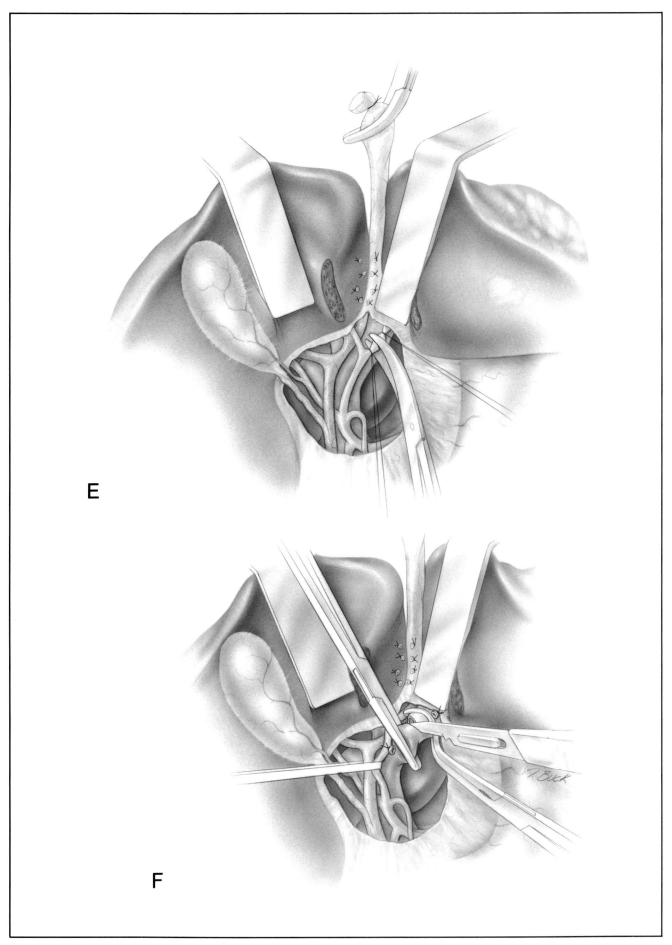

E

F

G Two bile ducts are shown arising from the left lateral segments. The base of the round ligament can now be divided, allowing access to these bile ducts and facilitating their identification.

H With traction on the round ligament and separation of the liver, electrocautery can be used to initiate penetration of the parenchyma. By keeping in the plane of the falciform ligament, damage to the structures of the left median segment is unlikely. The bile ducts from the lateral segments can be individually ligated.

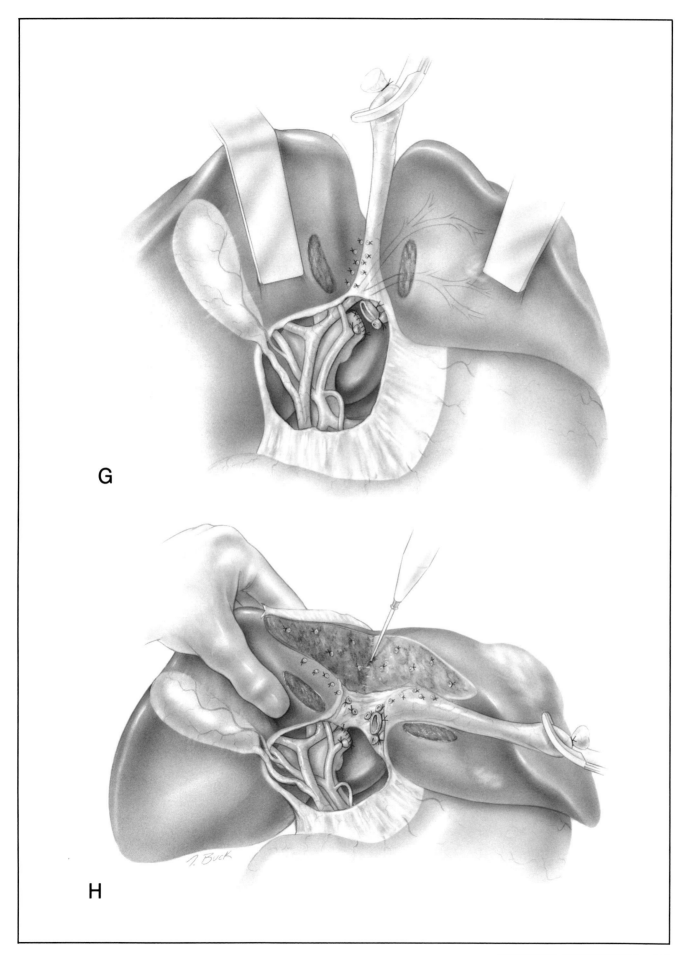

G

H

I Penetration of the hepatic parenchyma begins from the anterior surface medial to the falciform ligament and lateral to the round ligament. As soon as the base of the round ligament has been dissected, the left lateral lobe is gently moved over to the right side and its posterior surface exposed. Following along the line of the round ligament, electrocautery dissection continues between the caudate lobe and the left lateral segments. The triangular ligament has already been dissected, and this dissection continues cranially until the left lateral hepatic vein is visualized.

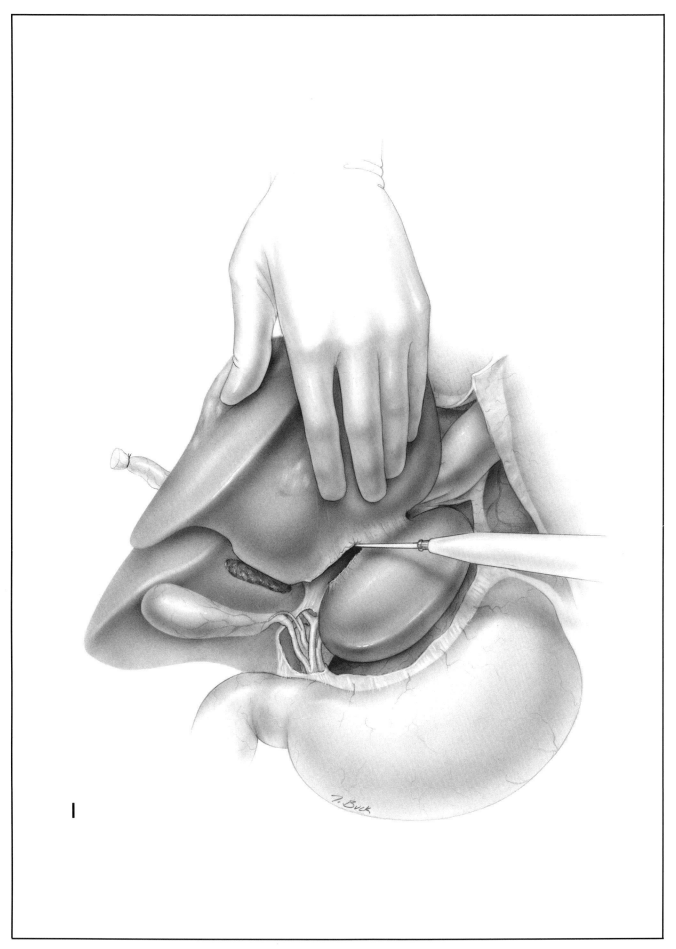

I

J

With complete mobilization of the left lateral segment by dissection of its posterior surface, the left lateral hepatic vein can be isolated, encircled, and safely disconnected. To find the right layer between the left median hepatic vein and the left lateral hepatic vein, a blunt, curved clamp can be gently passed from above, widening the natural fissure that exists between these two structures. The tip of the clamp can guide the dissection toward the posterior surface until it can be palpated emerging at the left side of the cava. A tape can be slung around the left lateral vein at this point.

Once the parenchymal dissection has been completed, the entire left lateral segment is mobilized away from its attachment to the left lateral hepatic vein. With this exposure, it is relatively easy (and safe) to clamp this hepatic vein and complete the removal of the left lateral segment. The orifice at the inferior vena cava is suture-ligated with a running 4-0 monofilament suture on an atraumatic needle. The cut surface is examined thoroughly in order to avoid hemorrhaging or bile leakage. Additional mattress sutures can be placed, using the falciform ligament as a pledget. The cut surface of the liver should be drained in case of reactionary bleeding or bile leakage.

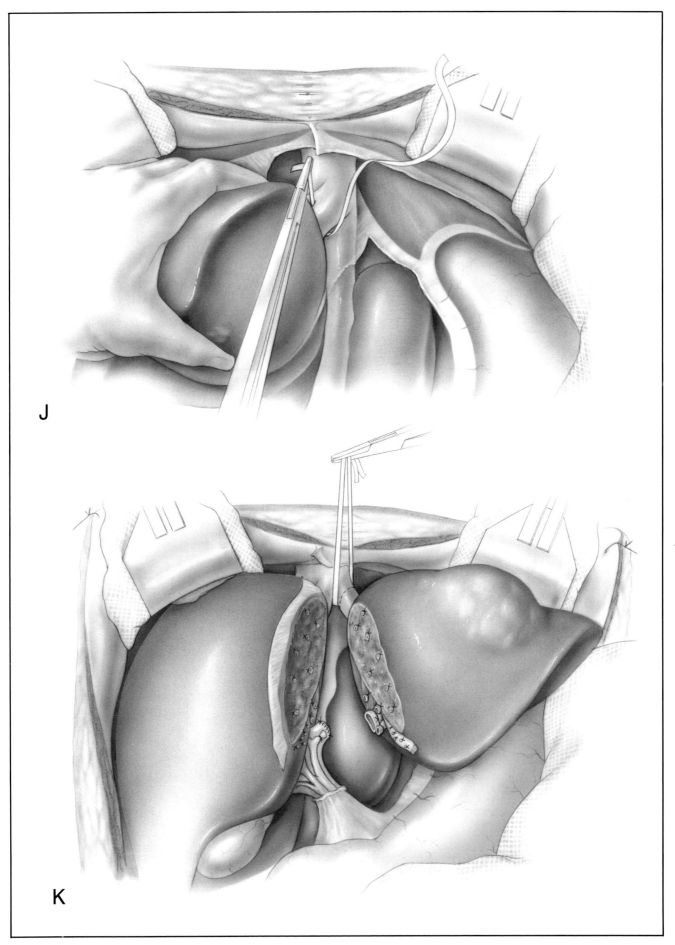

J

K

CHAPTER II

Liver Transplantation

Liver transplantation has emerged as an effective treatment for liver failure for a variety of liver diseases in the adult. Several thousand liver transplantations are done annually, with increasing frequency and steadily improving results. Chronic active hepatitis, primary biliary cirrhosis, and sclerosing cholangitis are well-accepted indications. Yet, the most frequent cause of liver cirrhosis is alcohol-induced hepatitis, which is accepted as an indication for liver transplantation, provided the potential recipient has abstained from alcohol for a reasonable amount of time (more than 3 to 6 months) and still has progressive liver disease. Furthermore, patient compliance, psychosocial background, and the presumed likelihood of continued abstention are additional factors in the selection of these patients for liver transplant. It is estimated that between 20 to 40 liver transplants are performed per 1 million people within the populations of Europe and North America, and about 50 percent of all transplants are performed for this disease. Indications for malignant diseases are questionable, although small primary cancers in patients with end-stage liver cirrhosis *are* curable by liver transplantation, provided there is no extrahepatic tumor involvement. Thus, the demand for cadaveric donor organs will steadily increase, and it is, therefore, mandatory to improve organ procurement and distribution whenever possible.

Concurrently, heart, pancreas, small bowel, and even cluster transplants are being performed more commonly, and the demand for these organs is increasing. Each donor, therefore, should become a multiorgan donor, and the surgical procedures should take this development into account. To date, standard transplants include the transplantation of kidneys, liver, and heart. Procurement of the pancreas becomes increasingly more important, although not all transplant centers have yet embarked on this procedure. The present description includes the approach for kidney, liver, and heart explantation and refers to special chapters in surgical textbooks for procurement of the pancreas. However, simultaneous procurement of pancreas and liver should be performed whenever possible, and one procedure does not exclude the other, although some controversy still exists about the allocation of the celiac trunk. Preservation of the splenic artery and the gastroduodenal artery is demanded by pancreatic surgeons, while the celiac trunk and the common hepatic artery is required by liver surgeons as well. Being a vital organ, it is generally agreed that the most appropriate arterial graft should go along with the liver graft.

1 | Procurement of Left Lateral Segment From a Live Donor (Anatomic Left Lateral Hepatectomy)

Living, related donor procedures are being performed by a growing number of experienced liver transplant surgeons. Segmental auxiliary transplantation is employed in patients with acute liver failure, but living, related grafts are used as whole, orthotopic grafts in infants and children (using the left lateral lobe) or even in adults (left or right lobe). The risk of the procedure is dependent on the size of the graft being used, and obviously increases with the extent of resection. The transplantable graft should be kept as small as possible to prevent liver failure and complications in the donor, but still needs to be of sufficient size to supply immediate, life-saving function in the recipient. Removal of the left lateral segment definitely represents a well-defined type of partial hepatectomy, but with the removal of only 25 percent of the functional liver mass. The risk for potential long-term complications in the donor is minimized, since the procedure does not involve formal dissection of all the vital structures in the hilum.

To minimize the risk to the donor, the hepatectomy should be kept as small as possible; only the left lateral lobe should be resected in most cases. This limits the number of potential recipients, since only infants and small children could accept a graft of this size. Left lateral segmentectomy is therefore designed to serve as a donor operation only for a size-matched pediatric recipient.

The potential donor should undergo an extensive medical examination and psychosocial evaluation as well as the surgical consultation. Liver, cardiopulmonary, and metabolic disease present contraindications, and donors above the age of 55 years should be excluded. The procedure is virtually identical to that described for an anatomic left lateral hepatectomy (see page 106). The donor is selected on the basis of angiographically determined vascular anatomy, including a single arterial blood supply to the left lateral segment, either derived from the left hepatic artery or from the left gastric artery. Furthermore, the size of the potential graft should be assessed by volumetric scanning to completely ensure size-matching.

A

The procedure starts as for an anatomic left lateral liver resection. (see Fig. 106). The left lateral hepatic artery is isolated distally to the branch feeding the left median segment. If the branch is of negligible size, it is suture-ligated in order to obtain more length on the left lateral hepatic artery. Usually, there are enough collaterals to support arterial supply to the median segment, and excision for ischemic tissue is rare. Below the artery, the portal vein is dissected from its surrounding fibrous tissue. Caution is essential, since the portal vein is fairly nonelastic and a few branches to the caudate lobe and the posterior portion of the median left segment may be damaged and cause bleeding. Dissection usually starts at the level where the caudate branch can be identified, but all of the branches can be suture-ligated proximally and distally. Under all circumstances, the left portal vein and artery must not be damaged, and their lengths should be maintained as long as possible. Once these vessels have been isolated, the left lateral hepatic vein must be freed. Dissection starts at the posterior surface of the left lateral segment, following the peritoneal tissue of the round ligament.

Isolation of the left lateral hepatic vein is obtained by careful penetration between the junction of the left lateral and left median hepatic vein. From above, along the surface of the anterior wall of the suprahepatic cava, the tip of a blunt clamp is passed posteriorly and medially, controlled with a finger placed under the posterior portion of the left lateral lobe. The left lateral hepatic vein can then be encircled with vascular tape. Control, but not occlusion, of the afferent and efferent blood supply to the lateral lobe is therefore obtained, and dissection of the parenchyma can commence.

The parenchymal dissection is carried out meticulously and cautiously. Using the mosquito and clamp technique, only small portions of the parenchyma are dissected and immediately suture-ligated. The hand of the surgeon may exert compression on the remaining liver on the lateral side of the falciform ligament, but no compression is necessary to the tissue of the explant.

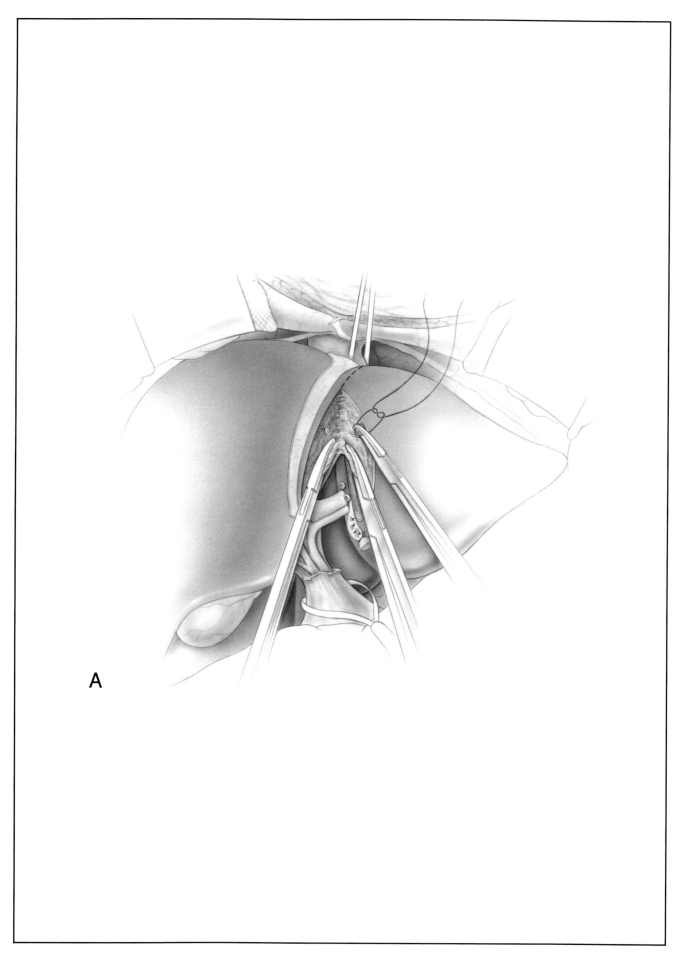

A

B With about half of the parenchymal dissection completed, the bile duct can be visualized at the base of the round ligament. The bile duct needs to be isolated carefully, and the existence of either a single duct or two small ducts needs to be confirmed. In most instances there is only a single common bile duct, although at this level the dissection is carried out directly at the junction of the anterior and posterior left lateral ducts. Once the exact isolation of the bile duct(s) has been achieved, the parenchymal dissection proceeds to the level of the left lateral vein. Bleeding from the cut surface is controlled by direct suture-ligation, assisted by mattress sutures along the cut edge of the parenchyma; great care needs to be taken to place the mattress sutures exactly, near the edge of the cut surface, to avoid areas of ischemia and necrosis. No mattress sutures should be placed near the left hepatic vein, in order to prevent venous obstruction.

C The isolation of the left lateral hepatic segments is completed. Bleeding from the surface is controlled, and the vascular pedicles are easily accessible. Normal circulation is maintained right until the excision of the lobe is performed. Before excision the back table is prepared, so that perfusion of the graft via the portal vein and flushing through the hepatic artery can be carried out promptly. Special vascular clamps are placed on the portal vein and the left lateral hepatic vein, and the artery is clamped with a soft bull-dog clamp; all three vessels are divided simultaneously. The transplant is immediately transferred to the back table, immersed in ice-cold saline and perfused with cold preservation (i.e., University of Wisconsin (UW) solution).

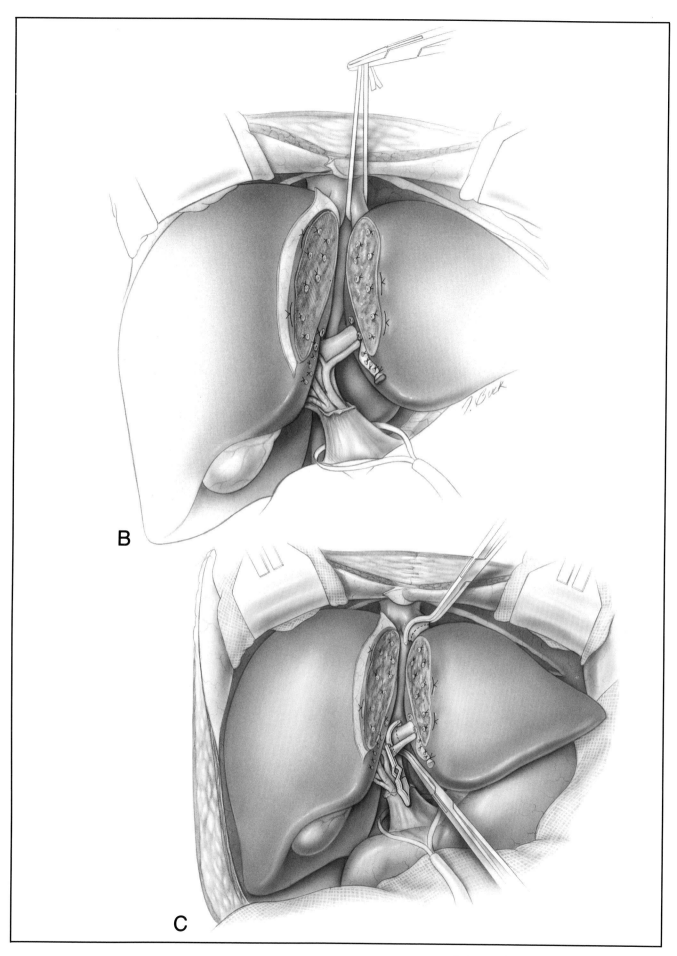

B

C

After removal of the left lateral segment, the orifice of the left lateral hepatic vein is carefully suture-ligated with running sutures of 5-0 monofilament thread, using an atraumatic needle. The stump of the left portal vein is also suture-ligated in the same fashion without compromising the diameter of the main portal vein. The hepatic artery branch is transfixed and suture-ligated. The cut surface is examined closely for minor oozing of blood and bile leaks, which must be secured meticulously. The surface is drained and the abdomen closed in layers.

It is of interest to note that, in our series, there has not been any necessity to transfuse blood, since no more than 300 to 400 ml have been lost from any patient.

The excised segment is perfused via the portal vein and, finally, flushed via a small catheter through the hepatic artery. Extravasations from the cut surface must be secured by detailed suture-ligation. As part of the procedure, the portal vein and hepatic artery must be extended with vascular interpositions. The size of the recipient determines the length of the vascular interpositions. The left hepatic vein may have to be incised and enlarged to a greater diameter, to allow optimal hepatic venous outflow after grafting. The transplant is stored for a few hours while the recipient is prepared for implantation.

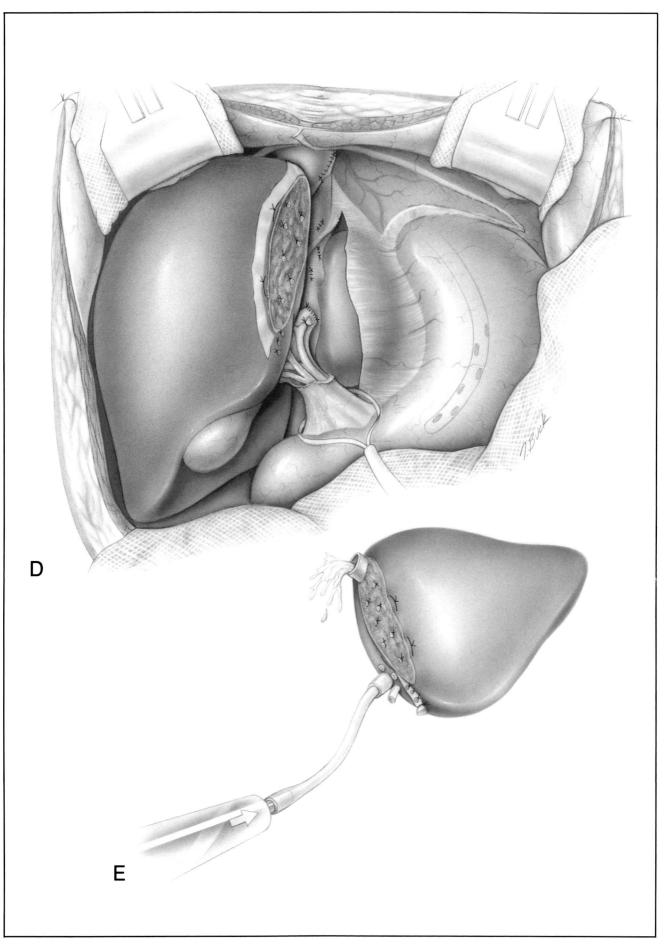

D

E

2 | *Removal of Infant Recipient's Liver*

Liver transplantation in children has become a standard procedure for a variety of liver diseases. Extrahepatic biliary atresia remains the most common indication, affecting 300 to 400 children each year in the United States. During their first three to six months of life, most of these children receive a portoenterostomy (Kasai procedure) to allow biliary drainage into an isolated loop of bowel and to prevent severe cholestasis. Although the majority of these procedures relieve the biliary obstruction, the vast majority of children continue to have liver disease, resulting in end-stage cirrhosis. Many require liver transplantation as the definitive treatment within the first 2 years of their lives.

The supply of full-sized livers in this age group is extremely low because of the low numbers of deaths affecting infants younger than 2 years. Adult livers are more widely available, and can be cut down into segments that function as independent, viable, reduced-size liver transplants. Today, the majority of children receive reduced-size liver grafts derived from the larger pool of adult or juvenile donor organs. The type of segmental graft the recipient receives determines the exact nature of the removal of the recipient's liver. Reduced-size grafts from cadaveric donors, which consist of the full right or the full left lobe, usually have long vascular pedicles (i.e., the portal vein and hepatic artery). Left lateral segmental grafts removed from living donors do not have a vena cava. This is very important, because their own inferior vena cava must be preserved.

The infant recipient of a segmental transplant is prepared in the normal supine position and appropriately wrapped to prevent cooling. Lines have to be placed before surgery, and often they must be placed with cut-down procedures. A double-lumen central venous line (Hickman line) is placed subcutaneously for postoperative nutritional support. The abdominal incision starts with a bilateral subcostal incision, usually corresponding with the scar left from the previous Kasai procedure. It is a rare bonus to operate on a child who has not had previous abdominal surgery; most infants present with significant adhesions and many collaterals from portal hypertension. With the abdomen opened widely, the subdiaphragmatic space and the dome of the liver need to be dissected first in order to reach the suprahepatic vena cava. Only sharp dissection with scissors or with electrocautery will allow dissections of the massive adhesions, which are collateralized with myriad blood vessels and require multiple (and patient) direct suture-ligation.

Once the dome of the liver has been freed of adhesions, the dissection continues from the right lateral side to gain access to the hilum. If the child has had a previous portoenterostomy, an attempt is made to isolate this loop, which will lead the dissection directly to the hilum. Approaching it from the right lateral side facilitates identification of the cava and portal vein.

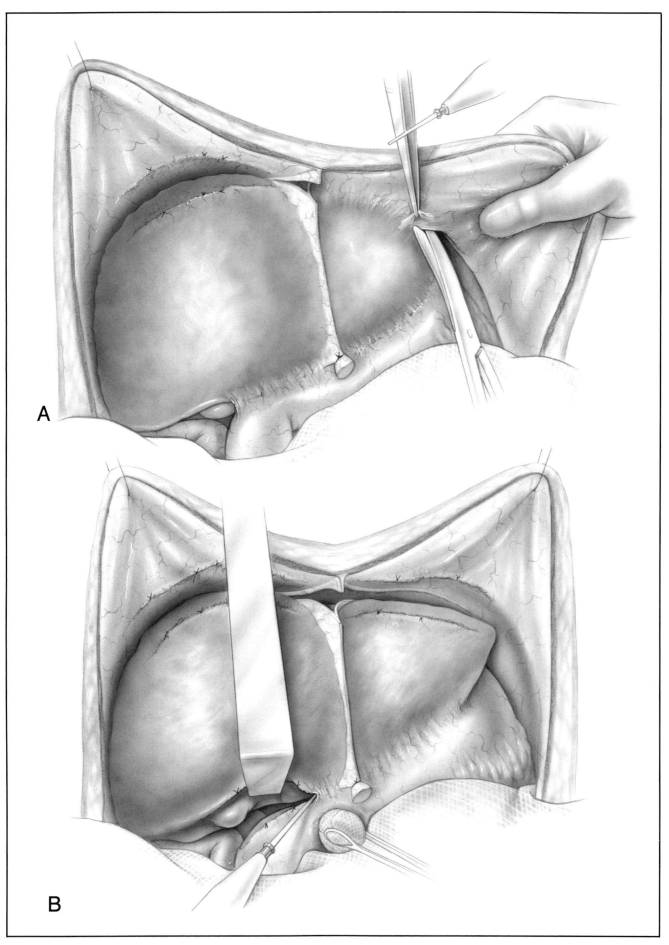

The Kasai loop portoenterostomy (if present) has to be released and the anastomotic site in the small bowel oversewn with interrupted sutures. If the loop is more than 30 cm in length from the ligament of Treitz, it can be used again for the biliary tract reconstruction of the graft. However, most of the loops do not have sufficient length, and the intestinal wall is severely traumatized from the dissection procedure, necessitating partial-loop amputation. The loss of 10 to 15 cm of loop is acceptable, although all attempts should be made to preserve as much bowel as possible, since a new loop will have to be fashioned.

Once the old loop has been taken down, the hepatic artery and its bifurcation should be visualized and both branches ligated separately to preserve the common hepatic artery and its bifurcation, which, in many cases, can be used later for the arterial reanastomosis. However, the artery needs to be reasonably large to feed the transplant sufficiently; if there is any doubt, the graft should be directly anastomosed to the aorta with an interposition graft.

After division of the artery, the portal vein and its bifurcation are exposed. At this point, the hepatoduodenal ligament can be encircled but the portal vein is not yet disconnected. Dissection continues along the posterior surface of the left lateral segment to dissect between the adhesions of the stomach and the capsule of the liver. Once this is completed, the lesser omentum is divided and the caudate lobe exposed, which leaves the liver attached only to the portal vein and the inferior vena cava.

 The portal vein can now be divided at its bifurcation. In infants, it is not necessary to employ veno-venous bypass, since the portal flow is diminished substantially and massive collateralization has developed through abdominal or retroperitoneal adhesions. Occlusion of the portal vein in infants is not accompanied by massive intestinal congestion, and is, therefore, well-tolerated for quite an extended time (i.e., 2 to 3 hours). The dissection of the portal vein allows access to the inferior vena cava.

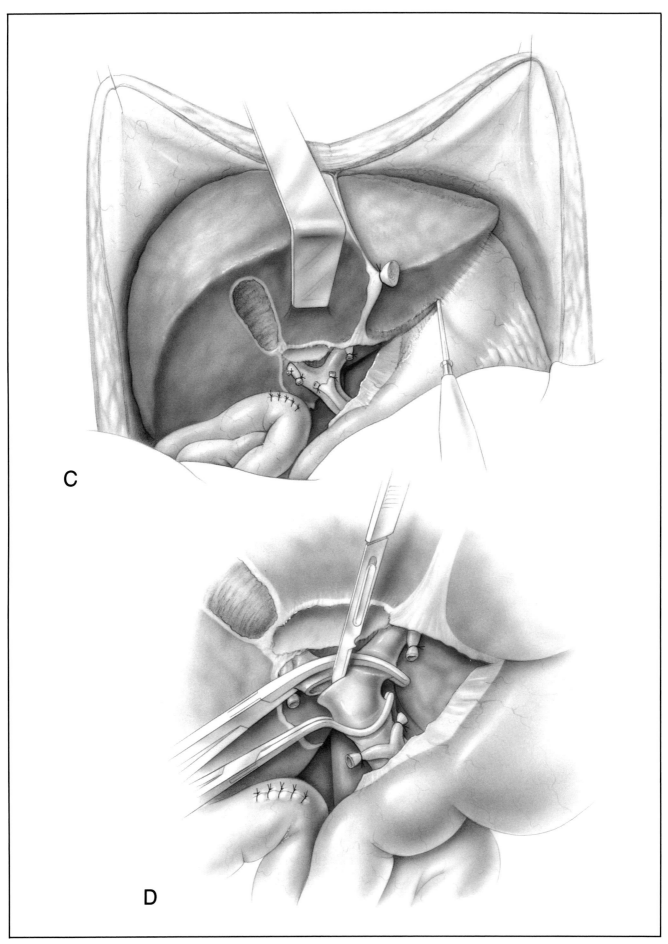

C

D

Since the inferior vena cava has to be preserved, all hepatic veins from the cirrhotic liver to the cava have to be identified and suture-ligated. The procedure starts at the right lobe. Gradually the right lobe is rolled over to the medial side, allowing access to the posterior surface of the liver and identification of the hepatic veins. This procedure is analogous to the one described for a right hepatic lobectomy and is carried out with the same technique. The advantage of disconnecting the portal vein is that the liver can be pulled up anteriorly, allowing identification of the hepatic veins without cross-clamping. The right hepatic vein should be clearly identified and carefully divided, then oversewn, avoiding narrowing the cava at all. Careful attention must be paid to all the accessory hepatic veins draining the posterior liver segments. The cava must not be injured nor its lumen compromised. Each tiny branch is painstakingly identified and suture-ligated with 5-0 or 6-0 monofilament.

 The liver is rotated to the left side and the left hepatic vein is identified. Again careful attention is paid to additional small hepatic venous branches. The vein is divided between clamps and the caval end oversewn with continuous monofilament. All minor bleeding from the retroperitoneum must be completely controlled.

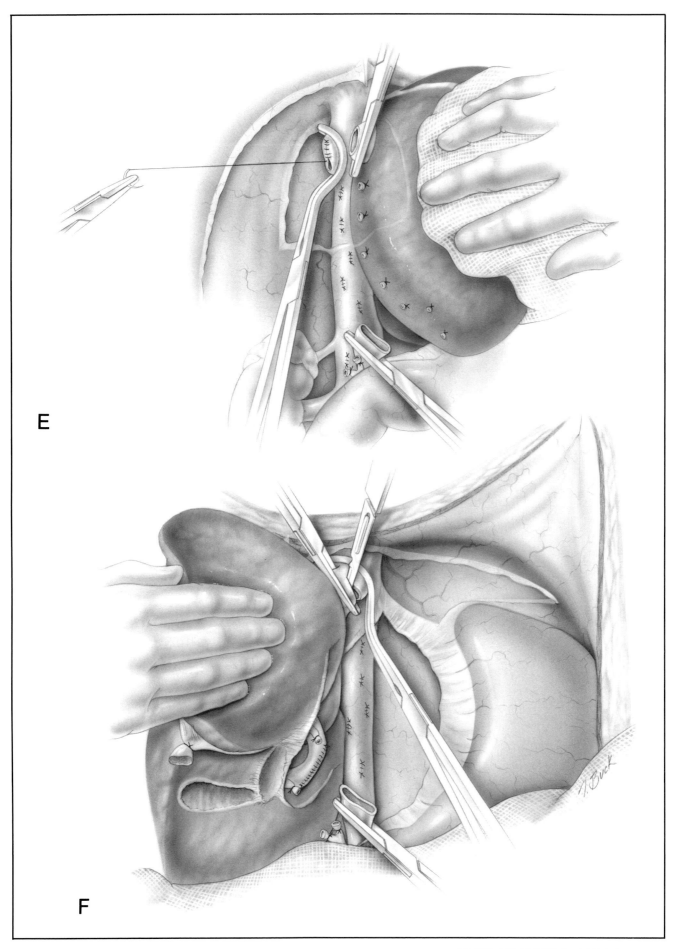

E

F

g The diseased liver is removed. The orifices of the right hepatic and left hepatic veins are oversewn and the cava is isolated between two clamps, positioned directly below the diaphragm and above the entrance of the renal veins. The following step is most important: a large triangular incision is prepared on the anterior surface of the cava, close to the upper subdiaphragmatic clamp. Part of the hepatic venous complex can be used for this orifice, which must be large enough to allow for maximal hepatic venous outflow. In particular, postoperatively, the opening of the diaphragmatic hiatus during inspiration will facilitate hepatic venous drainage almost directly into the right atrium.

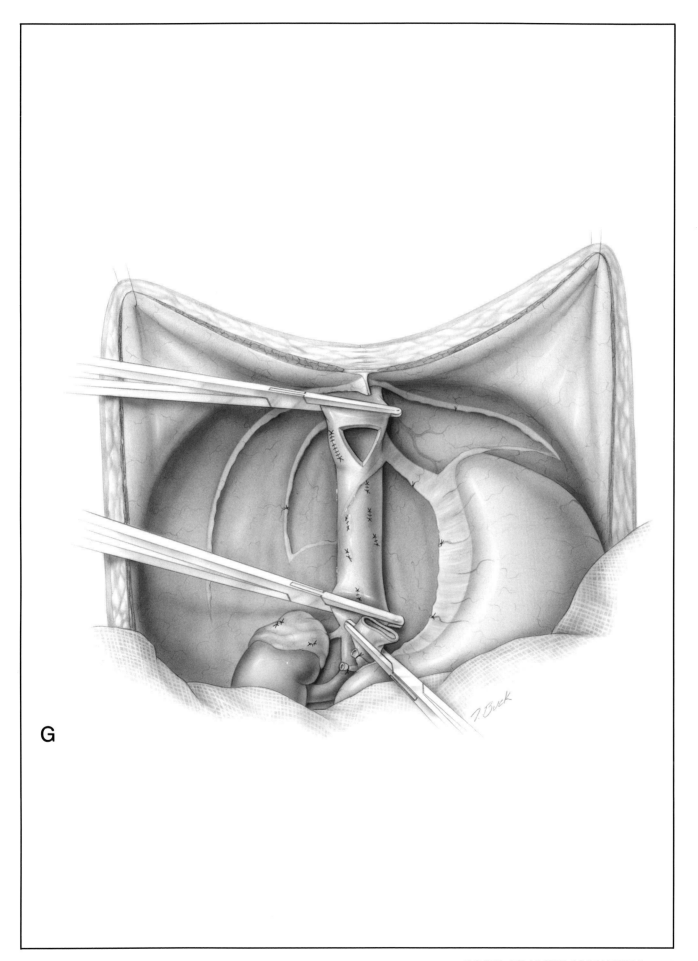

G

3 | *Implantation of the Donor Graft*

A The vascular pedicles of the portal vein and the left lateral hepatic artery have to be extended by an interposition graft of the donor's saphenous vein. Alternatively, a cryopreserved cadaveric saphenous vein can be used.

    The implantation of the segmental donor graft taken from a living donor should start with end-to-side anastomoses between the left lateral hepatic vein and the triangular incision of the anterior vena cava below the diaphragm. Sutures are placed at each corner of the triangular opening and at the corresponding positions of the graft. It must be remembered that the donor graft will be slightly rotated to the right side for its final position in the subdiaphragmatic space, and this should be taken into account when this anastomosis is performed. The anastomosis is completed with a continuous monofilament absorbable (PDS) suture on an atraumatic needle.

B With completion of the hepatic vein-cava anastomosis, a curved arterial clamp is placed on the left lateral hepatic vein directly above the anastomosis. The clamps on the cava are removed, restoring caval flow to the heart, and any leaks in the anastomosis secured.

    The portal vein reconstruction is completed next. With the interposition graft already sewn on the back table, the recipient's portal vein is dissected until the confluence of the splenic vein and superior mesenteric vein is reached. This is particularly important following a Kasai procedure, because the portal vein itself often becomes narrowed and fibrosed and a better flow can be accomplished by performing the anastomosis at this site. Because of the final position and rotation of the graft to the right lateral side, all vascular pedicles must be kept extremely long at this stage. The anastomosis is done with 6-0 monofilament absorbable suture. If both the interposition graft and the recipient's portal vein have a large diameter, a continuous suture could be used. However, if there is any doubt, this anastomosis should be done with interrupted sutures.

    Just prior to completion of the anastomosis, the graft must be flushed with 5 percent albumin solution through the hepatic artery to wash out the potassium-rich UW solution. About 250 ml of 5 percent albumin is gently injected into the graft via the hepatic artery and the effluent evacuated through the portal vein. The portal vein anastomosis is completed and the clamps released from the portal vein and the hepatic vein. With a living, related graft, there is usually excellent homogenous perfusion of the entire liver segment, and the low-pressure perfusion allows for easy control of any bleeding from the cut surface.

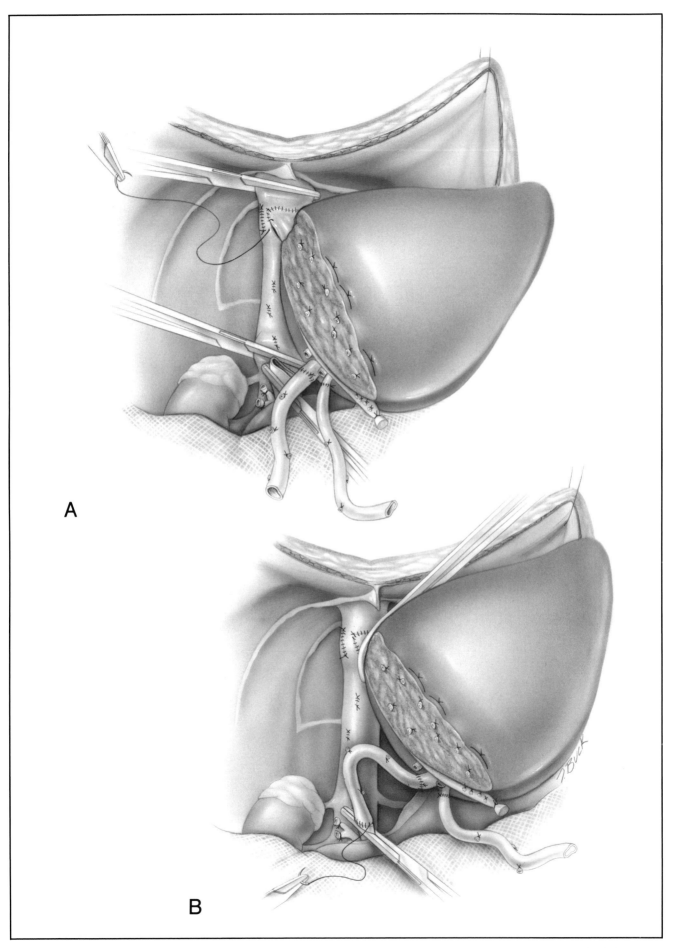

A

B

Reconstruction of the hepatic artery remains the final, most important step in maintaining a viable transplant, since postoperative arterial thrombosis almost guarantees graft failure. The artery must be handled very carefully and there must not be any tension on the anastomosis. Slight damage to the intima results in thrombus formation, thrombosis of the graft, ischemic breakdown of the biliary anastomosis, and graft loss. If the recipient's own hepatic artery is too small, the arterial reconstruction to the graft should arise directly from the infrarenal aorta. This is identified by palpating the aorta through the posterior peritoneum adjacent to the ligament of Treitz. A tunnel can be prepared to the graft from the anterior surface of the aorta, usually anterior to the renal veins and below the pancreas and the duodenum. The hepatic artery (or reconstructed artery with saphenous vein) can be pulled through this tunnel, taking great care not to cause twisting of the vein. After placing a Satinsky (curved vascular) clamp on the aorta, a small vertical arteriotomy is made in the aorta. The anastomosis is completed with 5-0 or 6-0 monofilament suture and is covered with a layer of peritoneum.

 Reconstruction of the biliary anastomosis is performed through a direct anastomosis between the left lateral hepatic duct(s) and an isolated loop of jejunum, which is brought up through a retrocolic opening. The loop is placed carefully in an isoperistaltic position without tension. A small incision is made on the antimesenteric side of the jejunum and the anastomosis is performed with interrupted 5-0 monofilament absorbable suture. If two ducts are present, both have to be anastomosed individually through separate incisions in the jejunal loop. Part of the loop will fill the right subdiaphragmatic space. Although the anastomoses are extremely small, we have not found that stenting carries any advantage. Note that the portal vein and the hepatic artery have a slightly curved shape in order to avoid any kinking through stretching or displacement of the liver. The natural anterior position of the left lateral segment graft has not given rise to hemodynamic problems. The anastomoses and the cut surface of the liver are drained and the abdomen closed.

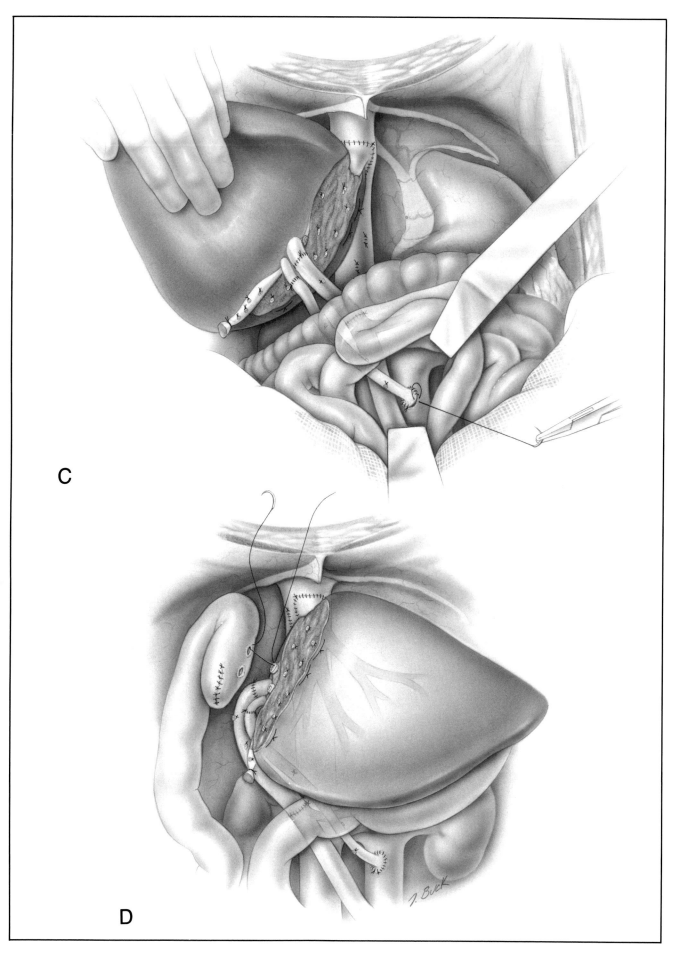

C

D

4 | Reduced Cadaver Donor Liver Graft for Infant Recipient

A

An adult cadaveric liver is harvested in the routine manner, preserving adequate lengths of the cava above and below the liver and maintaining long vascular pedicles. The portal vein is preserved to the junction of the splenic vein and the superior mesenteric vein, unless the pancreas is also removed for transplantation when the portal vein is cut at the junction of the coronary vein. The distal portal vein stays with the pancreatic graft. The hepatic artery is preserved in continuity with the celiac trunk on an aortic patch. The gastroduodenal artery and the splenic artery are ligated, as is the left gastric artery. (In cases of pancreas and liver procurement, the celiac trunk remains with the liver graft, while the superior mesenteric artery and the splenic artery stay with the pancreatic graft.)

The gallbladder is removed completely and the cystic artery ligated. The common duct is identified carefully and divided at the level of the cystic duct. If the graft was perfused with UW solution, bench dissection can be carried out safely, since this solution allows extended periods of cold ischemic time above 10 hours.

B

To procure the entire left hepatic lobe as a reduced-size graft, the common duct is isolated toward the confluence of the right and the left hepatic duct. The right hepatic duct is dissected and divided, and the orifice to the common duct is suture-ligated by 6-0 running monofilament suture. Underneath the duct, the right hepatic artery is dissected, isolated, and doubly suture-ligated. Care is being taken not to denude the left hepatic duct from the left and common hepatic artery. This allows for preservation of sufficient length of the left hepatic duct, since most of the common duct is being nourished by branches coming from the right hepatic artery. The right portal venous branch is identified next and divided. Its large orifice is suture-ligated with a running 5-0 monofilament suture with an atraumatic needle.

While all the hilar structures are being gently pulled toward the posterior surface of the left lobe, the line of dissection must be marked along the line of anatomic division between the main lobes. The line starts at the posterior surface of the liver between the confluence of the left and right hepatic duct, and runs through the middle of the fossa of the gallbladder to the fissure between the right and left hepatic vein, toward the anterior surface of the inferior vena cava.

The division of the lobe can be carried out by various techniques. Simple sharp dissection across the liver with a scalpel allows swift and accurate division of the lobes. The cava is also dissected with sharp instruments until the right hepatic vein is divided. The graft is flushed with UW solution to identify the leaks, which should then be meticulously oversewn under direct vision. We have chosen a combined approach, with sharp and blunt dissection, using the mosquito and clamp technique and identifying all vascular and biliary structures while dissecting the parenchyma. The dissection starts along the anterior surface and penetrates into the fossa of the gallbladder. The graft must be kept ice-cold for the whole procedure; most of the dissection is performed with the graft immersed in the water bath. Once the bifurcation of the right and left hepatic vein on the anterior surface of the vena cava is reached, the graft is rotated to expose the posterior surface. The inferior vena cava is dissected from its right lobe without suture-ligation of its orifices. Finally, the posterior surface of the vena cava, as well as the right lateral side, is freed of all hepatic tissue until only the left lobe and the caudate lobe remain attached to the inferior vena cava.

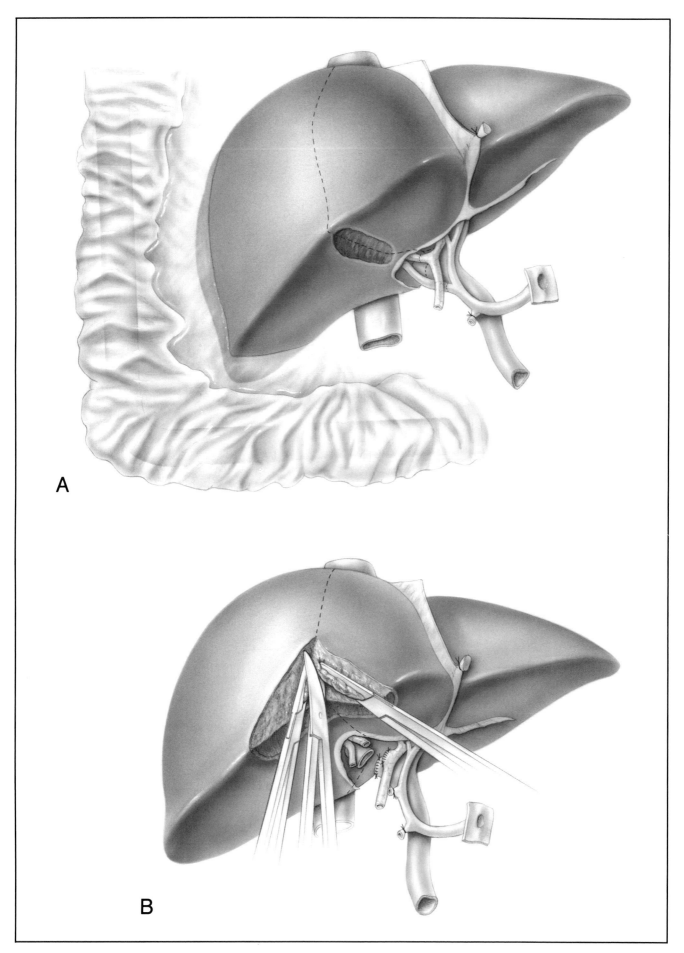

A

B

C
D
E

The dissection of the parenchyma is completed and all vascular and biliary structures along the cut surface have been suture-ligated. A few mattress sutures are placed along the cut surface, causing slight compression. No mattress sutures are placed near the outflow of the hepatic veins in order to avoid any outflow obstruction.

The vena cava of the donor graft is reconstructed according to the size of the recipient and the distance between the infradiaphragmatic vena cava and the suprarenal vena cava. Usually, the vessel is opened longitudinally and its diameter diminished to match the size of the recipient's vessels by resecting part of the cava wall. The cava is reconstituted using a 5-0 absorbable monofilament thread with atraumatic suture (4-0, 5-0, PDS) and its length adjusted to that required in the recipient.

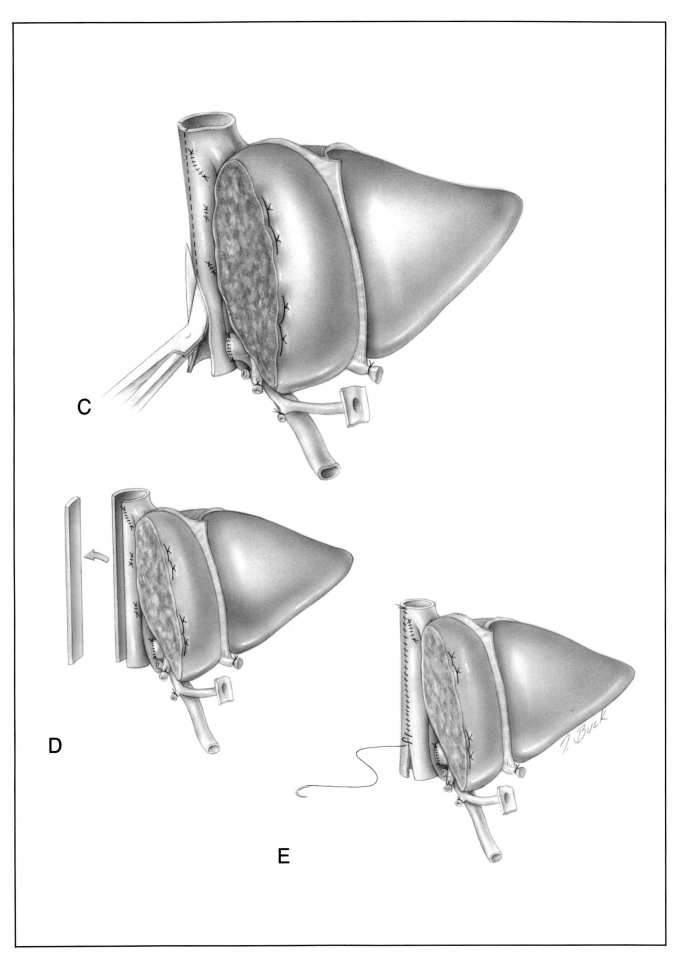

C

D

E

The recipient's operation for a cadaveric graft includes the total removal of the diseased organ with cross-clamping of the infradiaphragmatic and the suprarenal inferior vena cava, and the defect being replaced by the donor's cava. The superior anastomosis is performed first, with continuous suturing of the back wall and, subsequently, the anterior wall with 4-0 absorbable sutures. It must be taken into account that the graft will be slightly rotated toward the right lateral side, so that the cut surface lies in a posterior lateral position in the subdiaphragmatic space. The inferior cava anastomosis is then completed. The portal vein is next anastomosed in an end-to-end fashion, using monofilament absorbable sutures as well. Because the portal vein of the graft is usually twice the size of the recipient's own portal vein, the length and its diameter have to be adjusted accordingly. Often the anastomosis can be performed directly to the left portal venous branch, reducing the length of the donor portal vein to the bifurcation of the right and left portal vein. If the entire length of the portal vein is needed, the circumference of the portal vein has to be reduced to match the size of the recipient's portal vein.

The anastomosis of the hepatic artery is preferentially performed to the common hepatic artery, rather close to the celiac trunk, or, alternatively, near the bifurcation of the common hepatic artery and the gastroduodenal artery. Whenever the common hepatic artery of the recipient is small or when the recipient's liver had a dual arterial supply, deriving from the celiac trunk as well as from the superior mesenteric artery, we then perform the anastomoses between the infrarenal aorta and the donor hepatic artery. This decision can only be made intraoperatively, and usually a vascular interposition using a donor iliac artery graft must be used.

The circulation can be restored when the portal venous anastomosis is completed, though, if the arterial anastomosis can be performed fast and easily, we prefer to open both the arterial and venous flow to the transplant simultaneously. Obviously, vascular flow is better and more physiologic when both artery and portal vein flow commence simultaneously.

The biliary anastomosis usually requires reconstruction with the Roux-en-Y loop. The loop is isolated from the proximal jejunum and requires a length of at least 30 cm. Its proximal end is anastomosed side-to-end to the left hepatic duct. A small antimesenteric incision is made on the loop and a mucosa-mucosa anastomosis is performed, using interrupted 5-0 absorbable monofilament suture material. The biliary duct itself must be reduced in length until there is clear bleeding from the cut margin, even if only a short length of the left hepatic duct remains. The division of the jejunum in order to form the loop is extremely important, since the length of jejunum from the ligament of Treitz to the base of the loop must be kept fairly short to allow maximum absorption of bile and cyclosporin A. Cyclosporin A is directly dependent on the length of the small bowel, and early mixture of bile during its intestinal absorption is necessary.

All bleeding sites are secured and the abdomen closed in layers. The cut surface must be drained adequately.

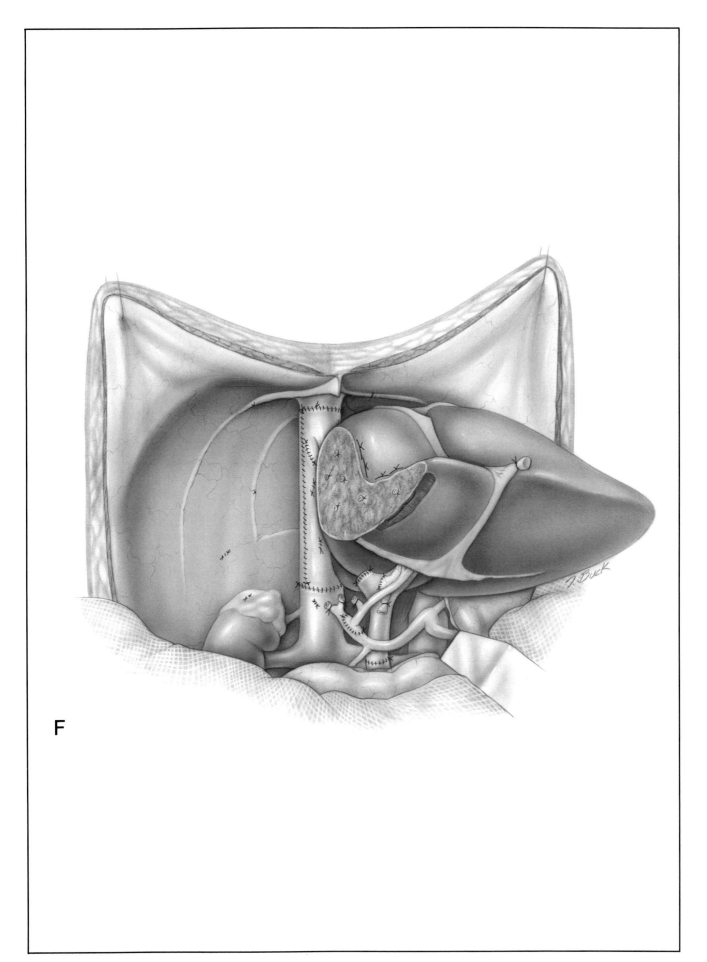

F

5 | *Removal of Cadaver Donor Liver for Adult Recipient*

The brain-dead donor is placed in a supine position with both arms extended, and then prepared from the neck to the groin for both thoracotomy and laparotomy.

The abdomen and the chest are opened through a midline incision, extending from the suprasternal notch to the symphysis pubis; strong retractors are necessary to maintain adequate exposure. In an obese donor, the abdomen should be opened through additional bilateral subcostal incisions to allow for better exposure. Usually, the procurement of the heart is done by the cardiac surgeon, who normally enters the procedure when the abdominal dissection is almost completed.

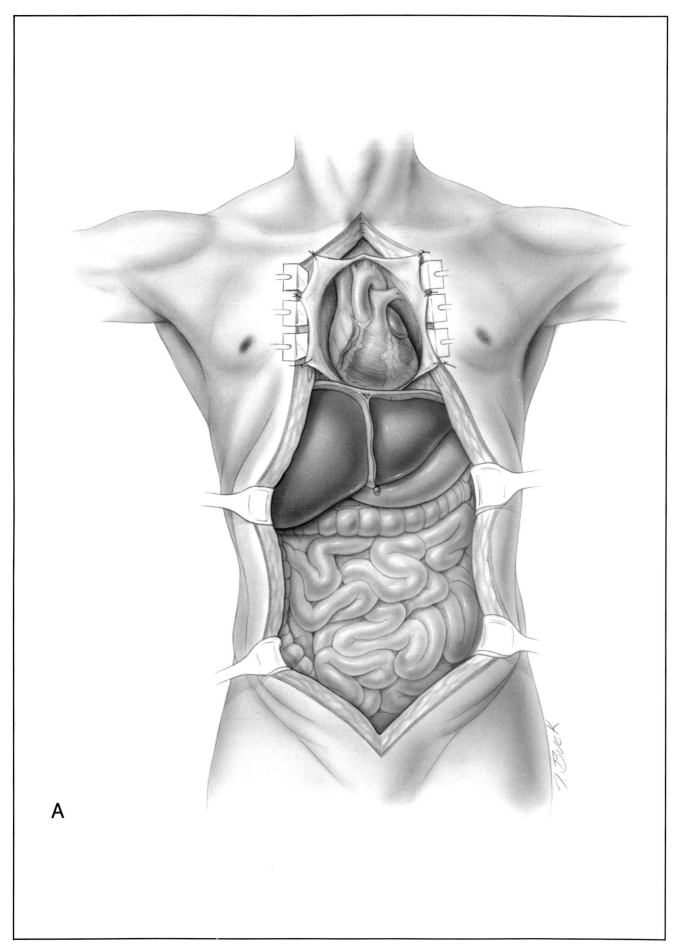

A

The abdominal procedure starts with full manual and visual exploration of the abdomen to exclude unsuspected malignancy and other disorders in the liver or elsewhere in the abdomen. Particularly, the presence of unknown primary or secondary tumors in the abdomen needs to be excluded.

The dissection starts with mobilization of the caecum, the ascending colon with the hepatic flexure, and the whole small bowel to allow exposure of the retroperitoneum, particularly the subhepatic vena cava from the renal to the iliac veins. The anterior surface of the aorta is exposed for its whole length to the level of the left renal vein. The inferior mesenteric artery is divided between ligatures. The superior mesenteric artery can be palpated when the whole small bowel is lifted over the chest; this artery is slung with a vessel loop. The inferior mesenteric vein is identified near the ligament of Treitz and is divided only when the pancreas is not being harvested. For pancreas procurement, this vein is used for the portal flush. The entire intestine is wrapped in a large, wet abdominal pad to keep it moist and facilitate its positioning. Care must always be taken not to compromise the portal flow in this part of the intestine.

The distal aorta is encircled and a perfusion catheter inserted and secured with very strong ligatures in a distal position, to ensure perfusion through the celiac trunk, the superior mesenteric artery, the renal arteries, and even accessory renal arteries, if present. Once secured, the intestines can be replaced in the abdomen.

The hepatoduodenal ligament is palpated to assess the hepatic arterial anatomy. Frequently, there is a separate right hepatic artery originating from the superior mesenteric artery. In this case, the right hepatic artery needs to be dissected individually, until its branching site from the superior mesenteric artery is exposed. In this situation, the harvesting of a pancreas becomes impossible, since the right hepatic artery needs to be preserved in continuity with the superior mesenteric artery. If there is an individual arterial blood supply originating from the celiac trunk, the superior mesenteric artery can be dissected and ligated. This will reduce the portal venous blood flow, but there will be sufficient blood supply to the liver through the celiac trunk.

For situations where donor circulation is unstable, rapid infusion through the aorta and the celiac trunk can be initiated as soon as the aorta above the celiac trunk has been encircled and occluded. This in situ rapid perfusion has been advocated by several authors and allows for safe procurement of the liver. However, all efforts should be directed toward maintaining a stable circulation, since procurement of the heart should proceed as well.

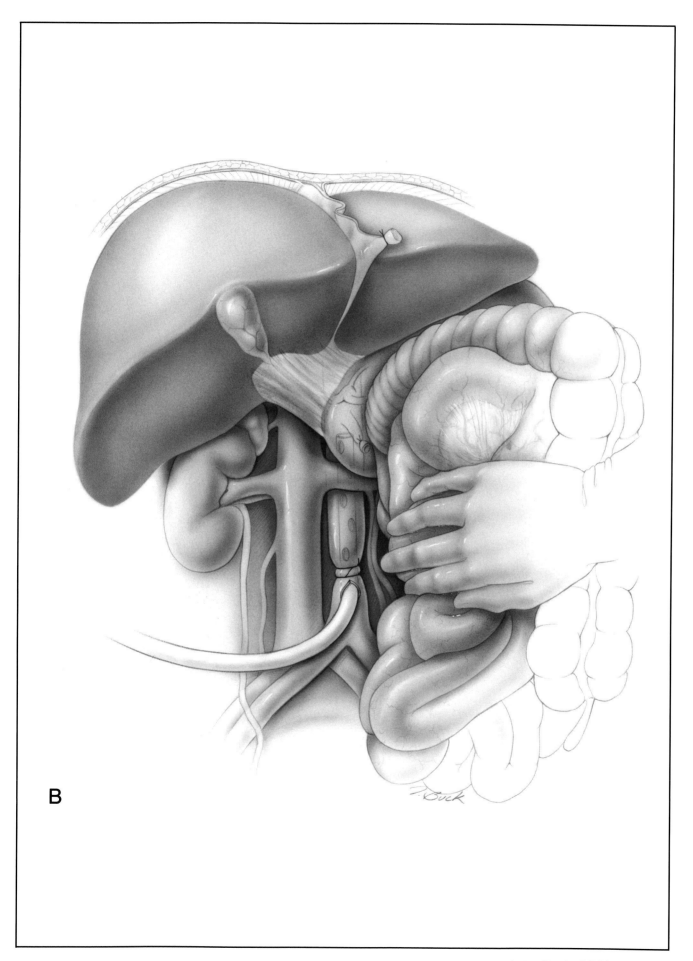

B

C
D
E

Provided the donor maintains circulatory stability, procurement of the liver continues with dissection of the falciform ligament, together with both right and left triangular ligaments. For all procedures, the liver is gently pulled downwards and can be moved to either side to allow exposure of the subdiaphragmatic space.

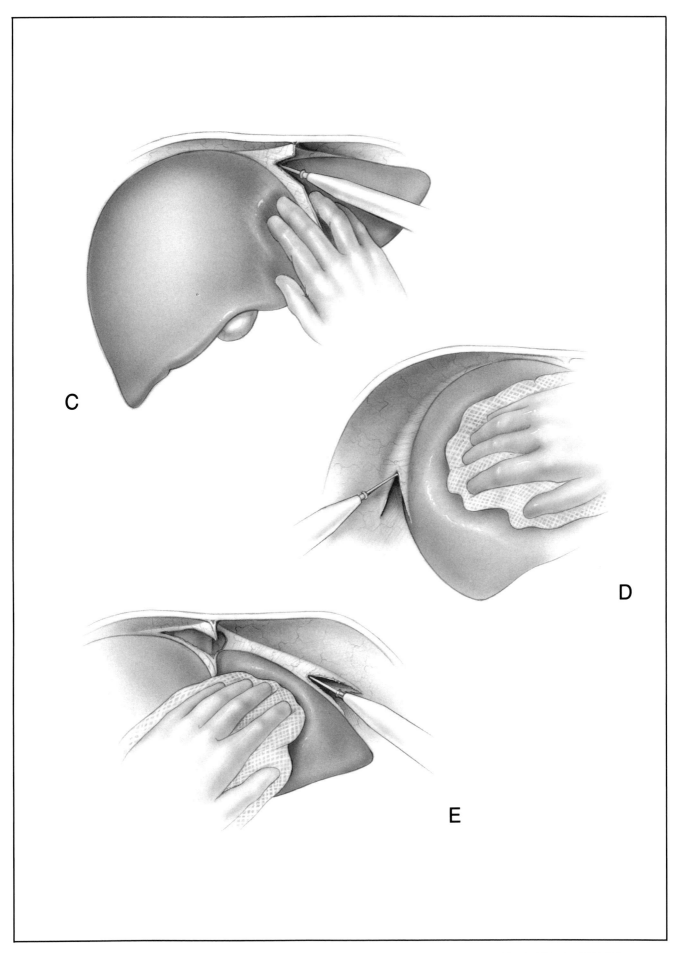

C

D

E

The dissection of the hepatoduodenal ligament continues with identification of the common duct, which is ligated as distally as possible—at the level where it enters the pancreas behind the duodenum. Once the duct is divided, the hepatic artery is dissected free and the gastroduodenal artery identified. It is carefully suture-ligated without compromising the lumen of the common hepatic artery. The course of the common hepatic artery is then followed, and the collection of lymph nodes overlying this vessel are cleared between ligatures until the splenic and gastric arteries are visualized. These vessels are divided and the celiac trunk is exposed toward the aorta.

The common hepatic artery is lifted gently to expose the underlying portal vein, which is freed of all its surrounding lymphatic tissue. The left gastric vein and the first branch coming from the pancreas are suture-ligated to allow the harvesting of a sufficient length of the portal vein. No further dissection is done toward the hilum of the liver.

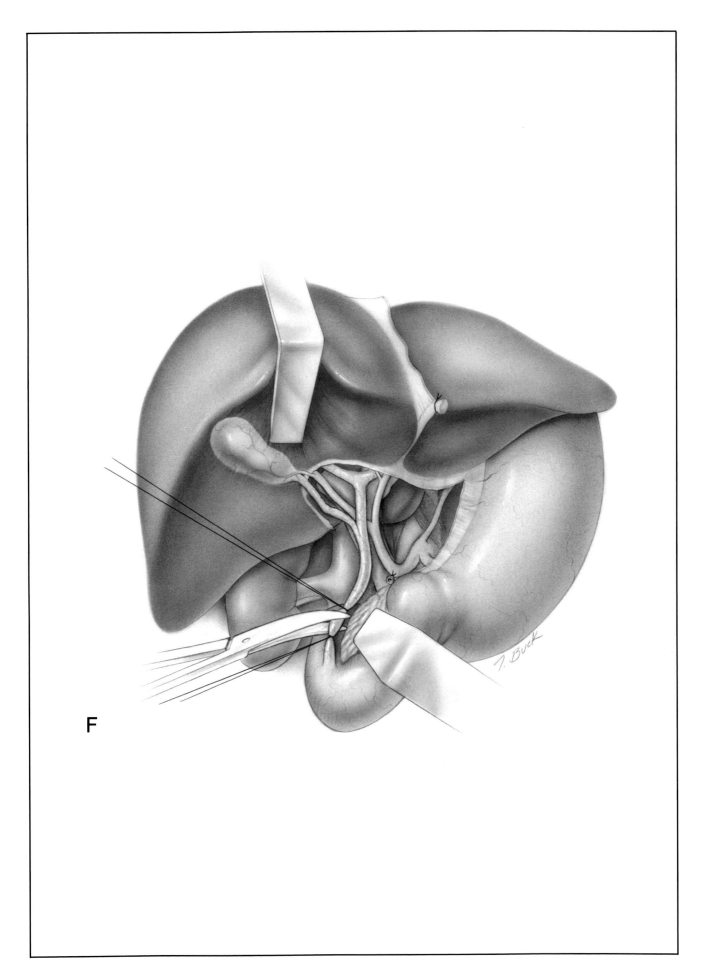

F

To accomplish simultaneous perfusion of the graft (arterial as well as portal venous perfusion), the portal vein needs to be isolated in its full, accessible length. When the pancreas is needed for transplant, the portal perfusion cannula can be placed in the inferior mesenteric vein. When the pancreas can be discarded, it is divided at its neck between two strong ligatures, which exposes the confluence of the splenic vein and the superior mesenteric vein. The superior mesenteric vein can be identified in the lesser sac, following its anterior wall, by blunt dissection beneath the pancreas, the confluence with the splenic vein can be found. The neck of the pancreas is divided at this level. A large Silastic perfusion cannula can be inserted into the portal vein, and the splenic vein is ligated. The liver is ready to be perfused.

If the patient is stable, the liver can be precooled with normal saline via the portal catheter while the supraceliac aorta is encircled and either ligated with a vascular tape or clamped with a straight vascular clamp. At this point, together with the aortic clamping, several maneuvers have to be synchronized and performed swiftly. First, the cardiac surgeons infuse cardioplegic solution into the heart and commence cardiectomy. At the same time, the supraceliac aorta is clamped and the formal liver perfusion via the portal vein and the aorta commenced with UW preservation fluid. The cava must be opened immediately, before venous pressure rises; this should be done in the abdomen as well as in the chest by incising the cava directly. Two large suction catheters are needed at this point to aspirate the vast volume of blood and fluid pouring from the cava. Finally, the superior mesenteric vein is ligated to allow further perfusion of the liver by excluding the intestinal circulation. The liver and kidneys should quickly be made ice-cold, and additional surface cooling should be accomplished by pouring more ice-cold saline into the abdomen. The perfusionist should always inform the surgeon that the perfusion fluid is flowing adequately.

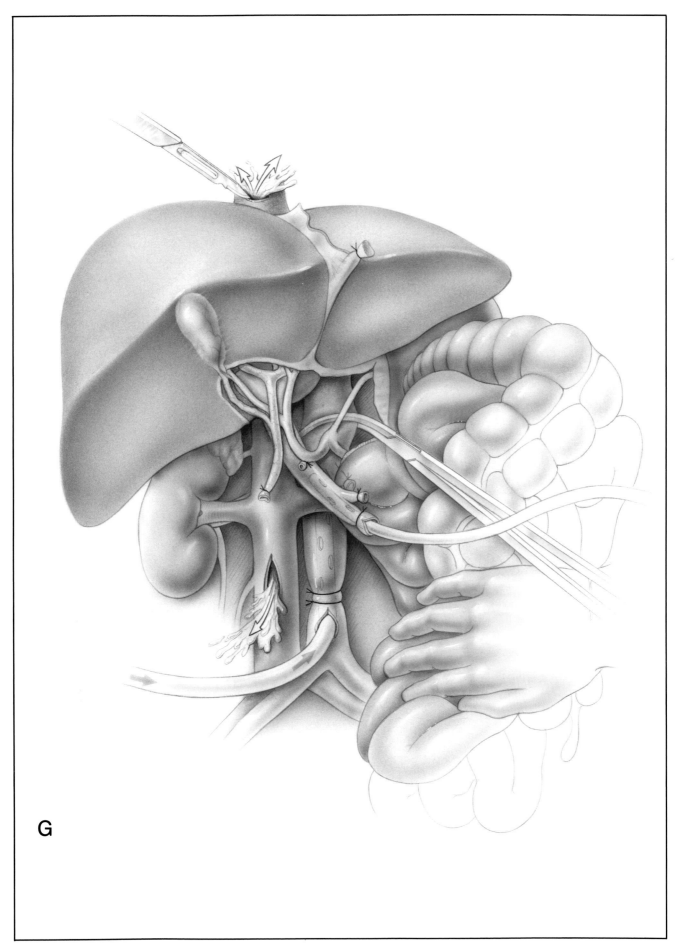

G

After perfusing 2 L of UW solution into both the aortic and portal cannula, the liver must be removed swiftly. It is mobilized by excising a cuff of the superior vena cava along with a margin of diaphragmatic tissue. The celiac trunk is dissected next, together with a small aortic patch, and finally the inferior vena cava is divided above the level of the renal vein. The perfusion of the kidneys can be observed through a vertical incision in the cava by examining the effluent of the renal veins; great care should be taken to provide a sufficient length of infrahepatic inferior vena cava, since only a patch of inferior vena cava is needed for a renal vein anastomosis. The final excision of the liver from the retroperitoneum completes the harvesting procedure, and the organ is stored in ice-cold UW solution and prepared for implantation. While suspended in an ice-cold saline bath, the vascular pedicles of the liver are examined. The hepatic artery is prepared and whenever necessary, suture-ligations are performed on off-shoot branches to avoid bleeding from the artery following reimplantation. The portal vein is prepared in the same fashion with careful suture-ligation of small branches, most arising quite proximally in the vein near the pancreatic site.

A cholecystectomy is performed, with a subserosal dissection of the gallbladder and careful dissection of Calot's triangle; the cystic artery and the cystic duct are ligated. An olive-tipped cannula is inserted into the distal common duct and the biliary tree flushed with normal saline solution.

The posterior surface of the liver is examined, and the lumbar branches to the cava are suture-ligated. At the level of the diaphragm, several small diaphragmatic veins enter the cava; these require careful identification and suture-ligation. A small margin of diaphragmatic tissue can be left attached to the suprahepatic cava, but all other redundant tissue must be excised. Following completion of this procedure, the liver is packed consecutively into three sterile Silastic bags containing UW solution and kept at a temperature of approximately 4°C. With this simple hypothermic storage, the liver can be maintained viable for up to 20 hours.

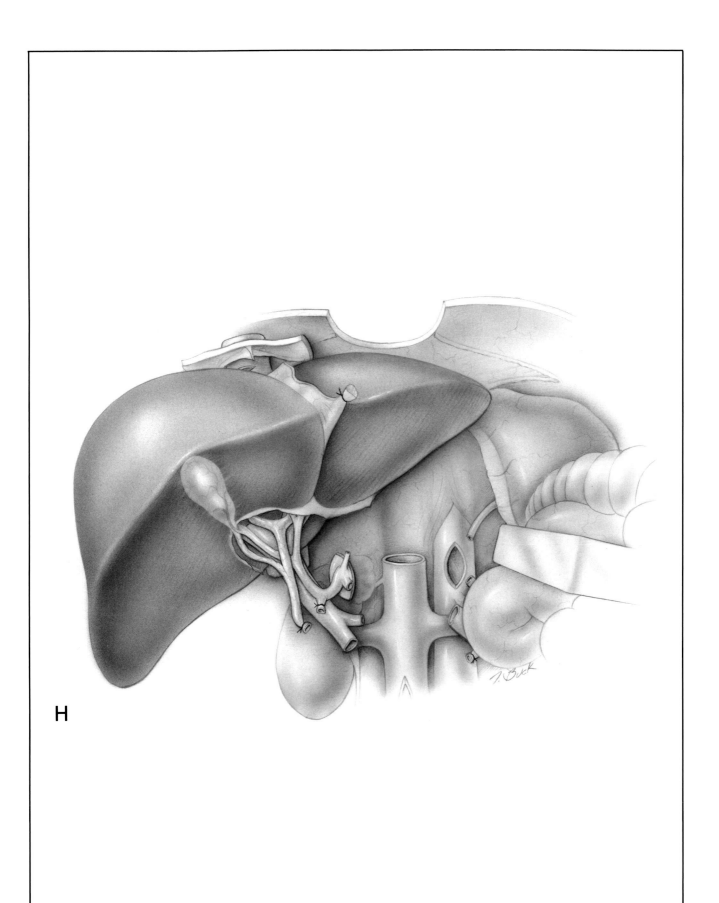

H

6 | *Removal of the Cirrhotic Liver*

The liver transplant procedure is one of the most difficult procedures performed in the abdominal cavity. In particular, removal of the diseased liver in the presence of portal hypertension can present a demanding situation for the most experienced surgeon. Many cirrhotic patients have undergone abdominal surgery for a variety of reasons, including cholecystectomy, splenectomy, portal caval shunt procedure(s), and biliary duct exploration(s). Multiple adhesions, undoubtedly formed from previous surgery, become integrated into a huge collateralization system, which may benefit the patient by lowering portal venous pressure and preventing esophageal variceal bleeding. Paradoxically, it is this network of collateralizations and adhesions that provide the most difficult obstacle in performing the recipient hepatectomy.

Collateralization, of course, occurs in cirrhotic patients without previous surgery. Periumbilical veins are widely dilated, and many of these require suture-ligation during the opening of the abdominal wall. It must be remembered that these patients have deranged liver function, and therefore coagulopathy, such that almost all of the vessels encountered during this procedure will have to be ligated — simple electrocautery will not suffice. Still, a substantial blood loss during the entire laparotomy and dissection procedure must be expected.

After the abdomen is entered through a bilateral subcostal incision, strong retractors are positioned to expose the subdiaphragmatic space. The falciform ligament is dissected first. Often electrocautery does not suffice to control bleeding (and occasional hemorrhaging) from the many collaterals within the falciform and triangular ligaments. Systematic clamping and suture-ligation is required to free the dome of the liver and allow access to the suprahepatic vena cava.

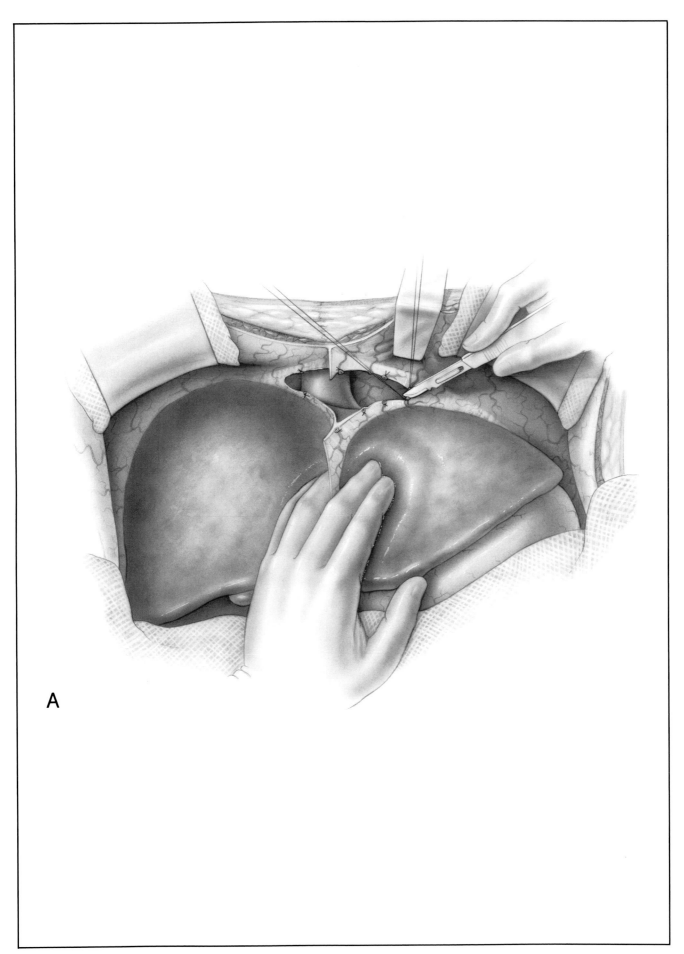

A

After completing the dissection of the dome of the liver, it is of vital importance to control the hilum and the blood circulation through the inferior vena cava. Before identifying individual structures in the hepatoduodenal ligament, a tourniquet should be placed around it to control bleeding from the hilum, in case of emergency. If possible, a tape should also be placed around the inferior vena cava, below the liver but above the renal veins. With these security measures in place, the individual structures of the hilum can now be dissected. Dissection from the lateral right side is preferable, because the bile duct can be identified first. Frequently, the bile duct is surrounded by large collateral veins, occasionally to the degree that a cavernous transformation has taken place, particularly if partial obstruction (thrombosis) of the portal vein has occurred. These veins have to be suture-ligated so as to allow identification of a section of the common duct of sufficient length. The duct needs to be followed close into the hilum and should be ligated as close to the liver as possible. If there has been no previous surgery performed in the hilum of the liver, the duct can be divided at the confluence of the left and right hepatic duct. The hepatic artery has to be identified and both branches to the left and right side need to be visualized and suture-ligated. Hepatic artery ligation close to the hilum should be done as early as possible, since it prevents bleeding from the surface and the capsule of the liver. The hepatic artery is gently retracted to allow visualization of the portal vein, which should be isolated from its surrounding lymphatics. Lymph nodes are usually edematous near the hilum, and most of these require suture-ligation; simple electrocautery is not usually sufficient to prevent continual oozing from their cut surfaces. The portal vein is mobilized for a length of 2 to 3 cm and will be divided high in the hilum.

Once the hilum is fully dissected and controlled, the dissection continues between the posterior surface of the left lateral segment and the lesser omentum, which harbors substantial collaterals as well. Usually, along the lesser curvature of the stomach, individual suture-ligations or running sutures need to be placed to control hemorrhaging from this site.

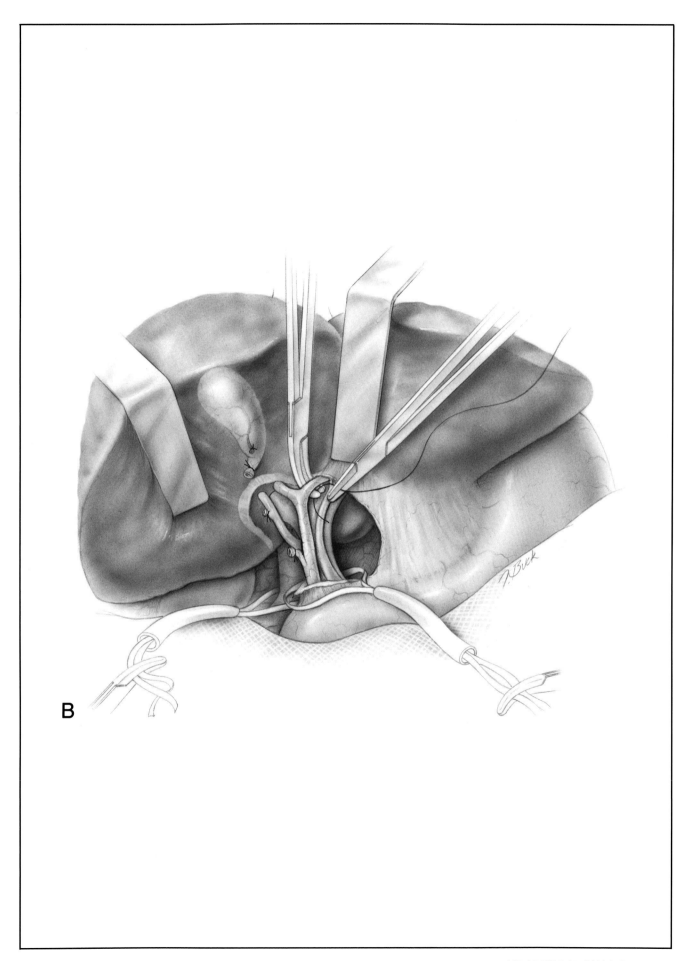

B

Whenever possible, the common hepatic duct needs to be isolated close to the junction of the left and right hepatic duct. The cystic duct is divided and the cystic artery ligated, permitting exposure of the proximal end of the hepatic duct. The left and right hepatic ducts cannot always be identified and ligated, but a duct of sufficient length needs to be preserved for a later end-to-end anastomosis of the graft.

Once the hepatic duct has been severed, the hepatic artery needs to be dissected to expose the bifurcation of the right and left hepatic artery and a segment of the common hepatic artery. Precise dissection of this area will allow for later end-to-end anastomosis of the graft's hepatic artery with the common hepatic artery of the recipient. Frequently in cirrhotics, the hepatic artery has gained substantial size and diameter and can be used for arterial reanastomosis. After the hepatic artery has been divided, the anterior surface of the portal vein can be exposed with careful blunt dissection by a peanut swab. The surrounding plexus of neuronal tissue and thick lymphatic tissue needs to be dissected and suture-ligated.

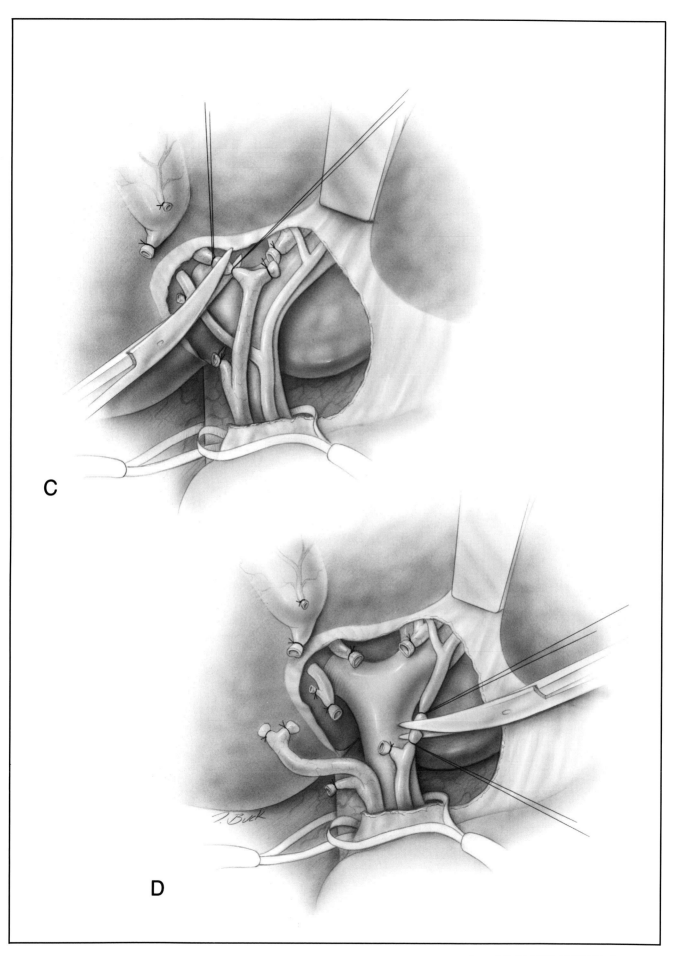

C

D

As soon as the liver is mobilized, with all the ligamental attachments and adhesions dissected, the portal vein can be cannulated in preparation for the veno-venous (decompression) bypass. The extracorporeal bypass diverts blood from the cava via the left saphenous vein, and the gut via the portal vein back to the heart, via the left axillary vein, and is driven by a vacuum pump. Full heparinization of the patient is not required. The saphenous and axillary veins can be prepared before the laparotomy to save time during this part of the operation. Large cannulae are placed into these veins and the bypass system connected with specially prepared Silastic tubing. The bypass can be started with simply the saphenous cannula connected, and the portal vein catheter connected subsequently. This system allows for substantial decompression of the portal venous system during the subsequent phase of dissection of the retroperitoneum and isolation of the infrahepatic vena cava. It is our preference to start the bypass at this point, because the disconnection of the portal vein allows for better exposure of the infrahepatic vena cava and the retroperitoneum. The perfusionist must monitor and adjust the flow during the bypass phase, keeping both the surgeon and the anesthetist aware of the flow conditions at all times.

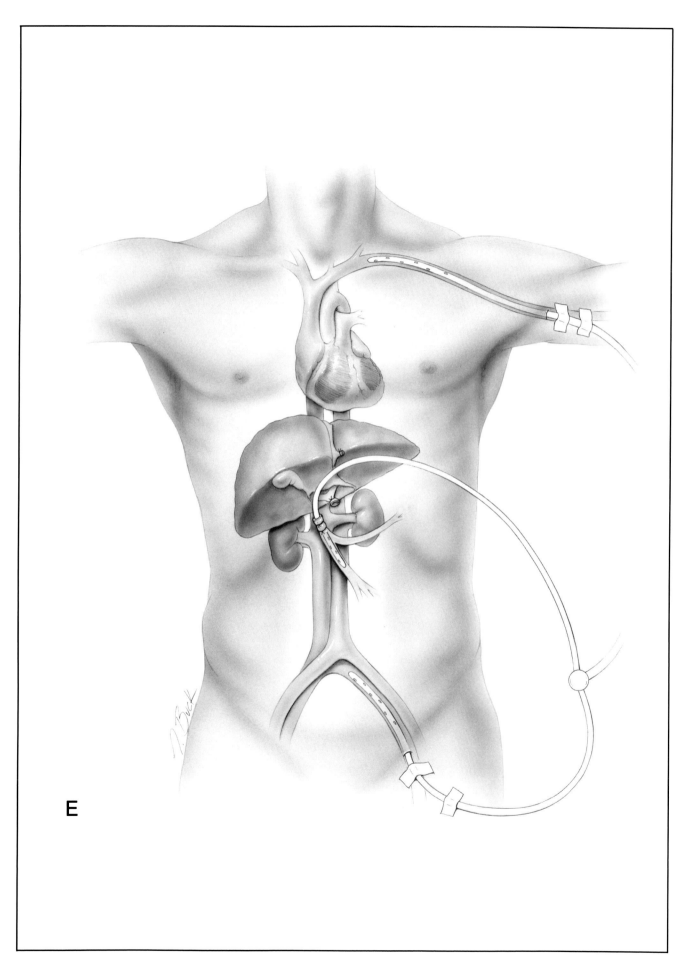

E

F   With the portal venous decompression bypass in effect, the inferior vena cava can be exposed and dissected. Numerous collaterals undoubtedly are present in the peritoneum covering the inferior vena cava. All these have to be suture-ligated before the vena cava itself is encircled. It is clamped with a straight vascular clamp above the right and left renal vein.

G   Circulation in the lower portion of the body is now interrupted completely, with both the portal vein and cava divided. During this time, the portofemoral decompression bypass will return between 2 and 4 L of blood per minute to the heart. With the infrahepatic vena cava clamped, the liver can be retracted and the retroperitoneum approached for progressive dissection of the peritoneum, which allows complete mobilization of the posterior surface of the liver as well as the inferior vena cava. Collaterals to the diaphragm and the retroperitoneal muscles all must be suture-ligated carefully.

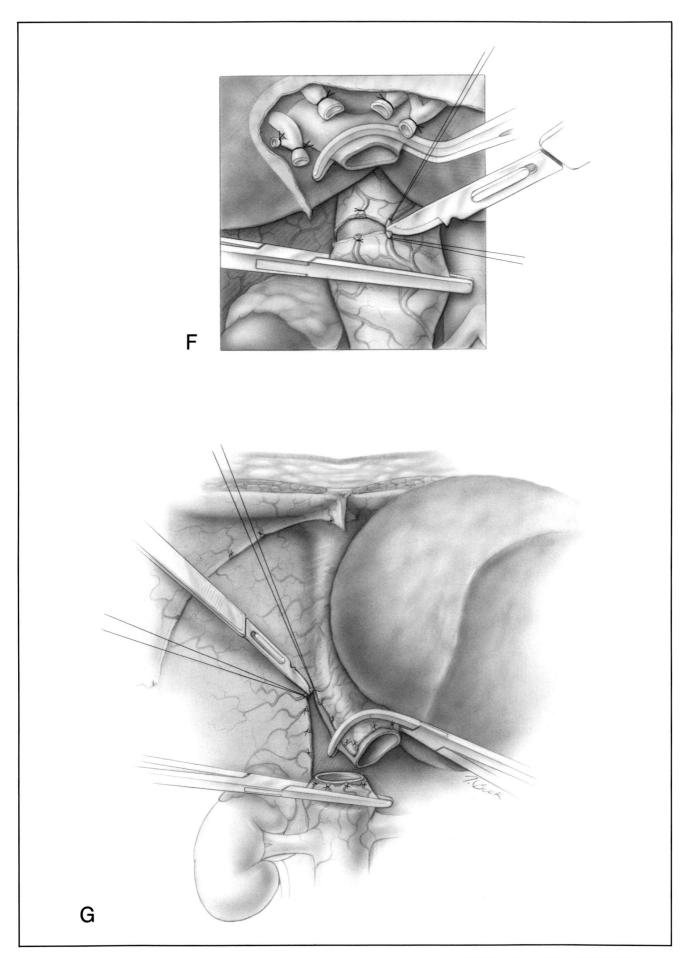

F

G

H Gradually, the liver can be lifted up anteriorly and the suprahepatic inferior vena cava can be encircled completely. A specially designed large curved vascular clamp can now be placed across the cava above the hepatic veins, perhaps including part of the diaphragm as well. The cirrhotic liver is then excised at the level of the right and left hepatic vein, leaving sufficient length of inferior vena cava for its anastomosis.

I Following complete excision of the liver, the retroperitoneum and the subdiaphragmatic space is exposed completely. All clamps should be reexamined for security and the bypass system checked. During this period, bleeding from the retroperitoneum has to be precisely controlled. Even with a "decompression" bypass in place, there is still a relatively high pressure in the collateral system, particularly in the retroperitoneum. Lumbar veins, as well as veins from the diaphragm and from the lesser omentum, have to be suture-ligated. Frequently, deep mattress sutures are required to control the bleeding from the retroperitoneum. Many times, plication of the diaphragm must be performed, particularly in the fragile area near the adrenal gland, which requires careful attention. With the veno-venous bypass system in place, the patient can tolerate cross-clamping of the cava and portal vein fairly well for at least 3 hours.

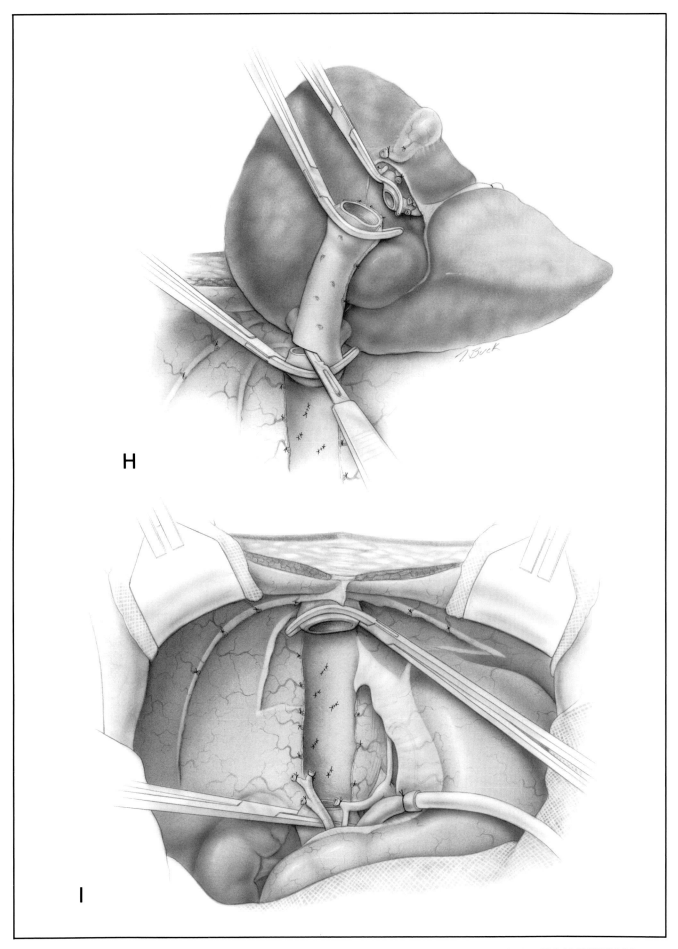

H

I

7 | *Implantation of the Adult Donor Graft*

After removal of the diseased liver, which can prove extremely difficult in some circumstances, the implantation procedure usually provides less of a challenge. Good size-matching between donor and recipient, together with strong retraction, ensures that the vascular anastomoses can be done expeditiously.

The procedure begins with the end-to-end anastomosis of the suprahepatic inferior vena cava. First, the back wall is sewn with a 3-0 monofilament atraumatic suture, after corner stitches have been placed. It is important to adapt the intimal layers of both vessels carefully, and to insist on excellent exposure, so that each stitch can be placed perfectly. The tension is maintained throughout and care taken not to stenose the graft's hepatic veins. The anterior wall is sewn in a similar fashion, with a continuous 3-0 monofilament atraumatic suture and the suture secured. The surface of the liver must be kept moist with ice-cold pads throughout the procedure to minimize warming of the liver.

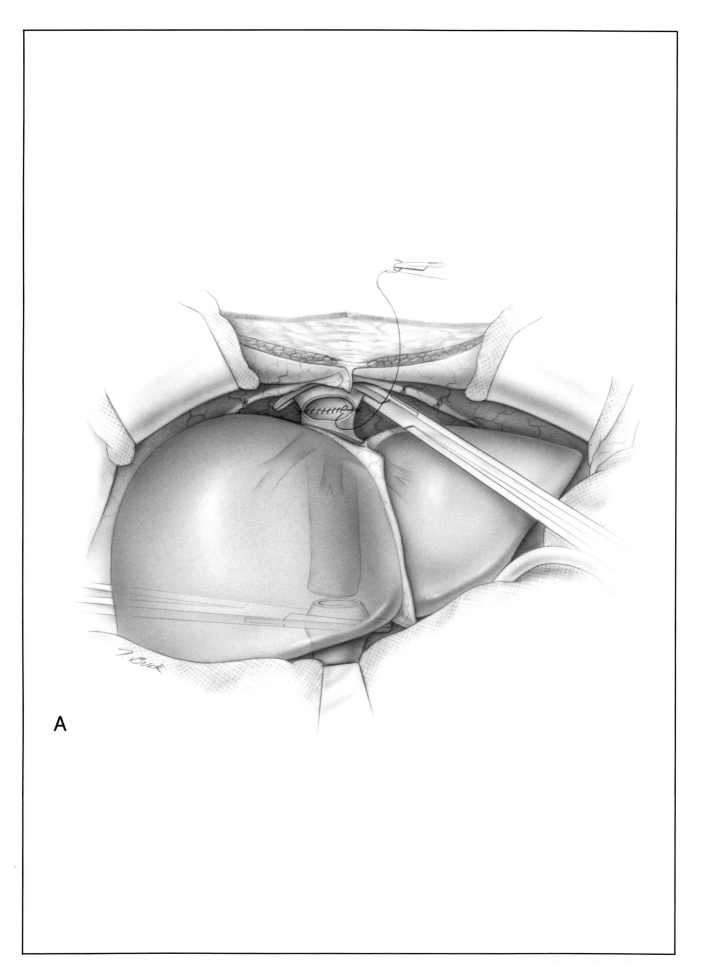

A

After the upper anastomosis is completed, the infraheaptic cava is anastomosed in an end-to-end fashion. After corner stitches have identified the correct alignment, the posterior wall is sewn first, with 4-0 monofilament running suture, followed by the anterior wall. Before tying the corner thread with the suture of the anterior wall, a small catheter is placed into the lumen to vent the cava by allowing evacuation of the perfusate just prior to reperfusion of the graft.

If the patient is stable and the portal veno-venous bypass is still running effectively, both the arterial and portal anastomoses are completed to accomplish recirculation to the graft by simultaneous release of the hepatic arterial flow and the portal venous flow. The portal vein containing the Silastic catheter is gently retracted and the common hepatic artery is exposed. This artery is then explored until its caliber is sufficient to allow for a large anastomosis.

There are two commonly employed techniques in reconstruction of the hepatic artery. First, an end-to-end anastomosis between the two hepatic arteries can be performed without a patch, provided the lumens of the arteries are of comparable diameter. The end-to-end anastomosis is performed using 6-0 interrupted sutures of monofilament nonabsorbable atraumatic suture. Second, the patch of the celiac trunk can be incorporated into an anastomosis in a end-to-side fashion to the common hepatic artery, near the origin of the splenic and left gastric artery. The recipient's gastroduodenal artery is divided or clamped and the trifurcation exposed as much as possible. A longitudinal incision in the common hepatic artery enables the patch to be sewn in place using 6-0 monofilament continuous suture on an atraumatic needle. Before completion, the lumen must be flushed with heparin-saline solution to wash out any potential thrombotic material.

After completion of the arterial anastomosis, the donor artery is clamped by a soft vascular bulldog clamp near the site of the anastomosis, and the clamps from the common hepatic artery and the gastroduodenal artery are released. Hemostasis is secured at this site. The bypass catheter is removed from the portal vein, which is clamped near its origin with a small curved vascular clamp. The portal vein anastomosis is performed in an end-to-end fashion after it is approximated in length and size to the donor portal vein. It is sutured using 5-0 atraumatic monofilament suture. Before completion of the anastomosis, a Silastic catheter is introduced into the donor portal vein, and the liver is flushed with 5 percent albumin to wash out the potassium-rich residual UW solution. The perfusate is evacuated by the vent catheter previously placed into the inferior vena cava.

Following perfusion with 2 L of albumin solution and careful manual squeezing of the inferior vena cava for evacuation of residual air, the cannula is removed and the anastomosis of the cava is completed and secured. The portal vein anastomosis is completed after removal of the perfusion catheter by carefully expanding the corner stitches and gently pulling on the running suture to complete approximation of the vessel walls. There should be no tension at this site and no stenosis. Simultaneously, the flow of the extracorporeal bypass is reduced to a maintenance flow of 500 ml/min and the upper and lower vena cava clamps are released. At this time, the anesthesiologist exerts a slight positive end expiratory pressure (PEEP), gradually increasing the pressure in the inferior vena cava. Bleeding sites from the cava are secured with 4-0 monofilament thread. Occasionally, small branches near the diaphragm start to bleed after removal of the clamps, but these can be controlled relatively easily because of the low pressure in the cava at this time.

Shortly after releasing the clamps from the cava, portal and hepatic arterial circulation is restored. Both clamps are released simultaneously, allowing for optimal initial reperfusion of the graft. Immediately following revascularization, warm irrigation fluid is poured into the abdomen to accelerate rewarming of the graft. All sites of bleeding now require careful control. Electrocautery suffices to control bleeding from the fossa of the gallbladder. Bleeding from the cut edge of the distal common duct is initially controlled by a soft vascular bulldog clamp. Bleeding from the capsule of the liver or the retroperitoneum requires additional electrocoagulation or direct suture-ligation.

While the liver is being rewarmed and gently packed with warm pads, the decompression bypass is removed from the saphenous vein in the groin and the subclavian vein in the axilla. Whenever possible these vessels are preserved and carefully reconstituted, using 5-0 or 6-0 monofilament suture. In the groin, prevention of lymphatic leakage must be performed by careful ligation of all identifiable lymphatic structures, and the wound drained for 24 hours. The wound is closed in individual layers.

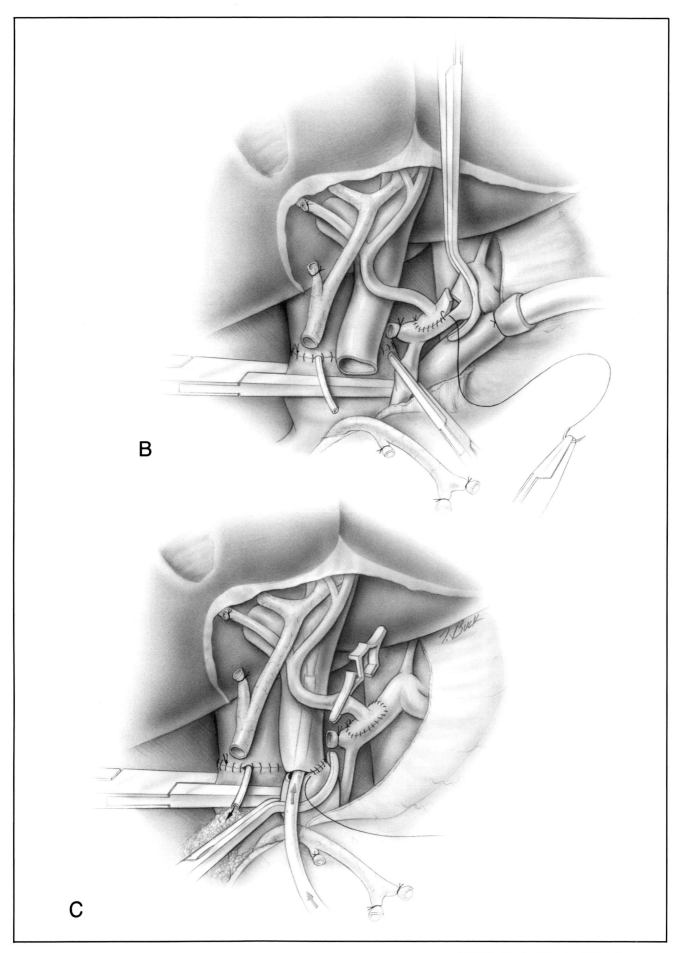

B

C

Reanastomosis of the biliary duct can be performed using a variety of techniques. An end-to-end, duct-to-duct anastomosis is the most commonly employed, but must be done without tension. The use of a T-tube is still debatable and depends on individual preference. It is important to assess the viability of the margin of anastomosis, so, on the donor side, the common duct is cut back until detectable arterial bleeding occurs. A mucosa-mucosa anastomosis can be performed, using interrupted sutures of 5-0 absorbable monofilament suture material.

A side-to-side anastomosis is perhaps preferable, but long ducts on both sides are necessary. The two ducts are placed parallel to each other and longitudinal incisions made in each. The anastomosis is completed with continuous absorbable sutures. A T-tube is optional. This side-to-side anastomosis is gaining more popularity, since it carries a low complication rate.

Finally, all areas are inspected and bleeding sites secured. The whole implantation field must be thoroughly drained, with drains placed above and below the liver on the right and left side. Whenever there has been extensive dissection of the diaphragm, or it has been traumatized, a chest drain should be inserted.

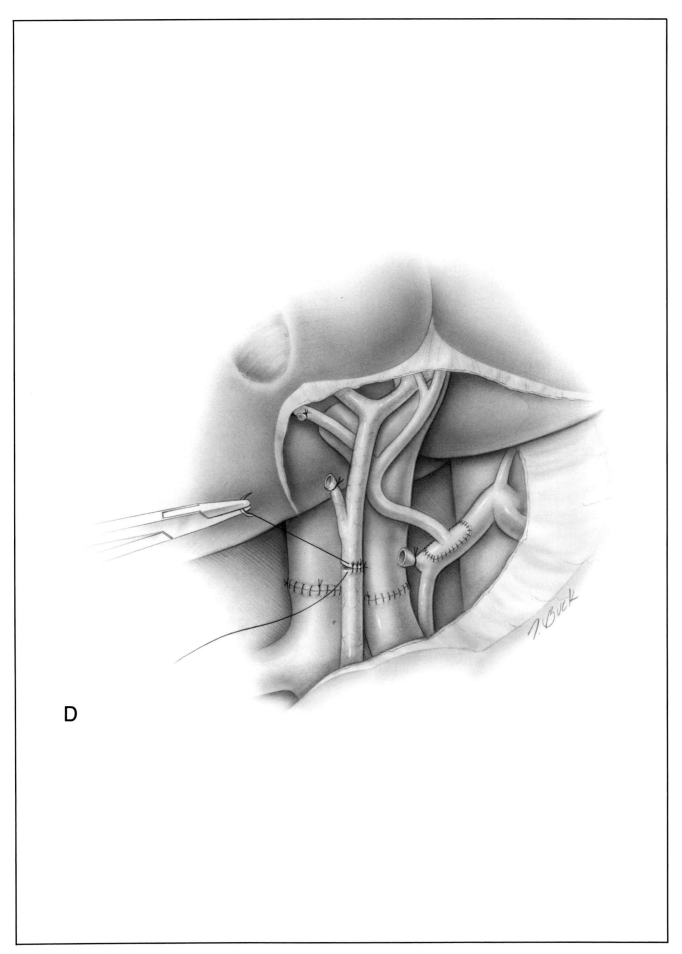

D

CHAPTER III

Biliary Tree Reconstruction

Malignant tumors arising from the confluence of the main hepatic ducts or common hepatic ducts form a distinct clinical entity. They present with painless jaundice in the absence of preexistent liver disease or calculus disease of the gallbladder or biliary system. Patients in their 40s to 60s are preferentially affected. The diagnosis is suspected radiologically by endoscopic cholangiography and/or percutaneous transhepatic cholangiography. Histologically, these tumors are usually adenocarcinomas of the bile duct wall that contain large quantities of fibrous tissue resembling a scirrhous carcinoma. It is this fibrosis that causes mechanical obstruction and leads to the clinical symptoms of jaundice.

The location of the tumor can range along the common hepatic duct, with a subjunctional site below the confluence of the hepatic ducts, extension into the right or left hepatic duct, or involvement of the junction and both hepatic ducts. The proximal extent of these tumors can only be assessed correctly with percutaneous transhepatic cholangiography. The surgical approach to these tumors is still controversial, as simple endoscopic or percutaneous drainage by stenting often relieves symptoms and may provide long-term survival because of the slow-growing nature of the cancer. Furthermore, surgical resection is often incomplete in the majority of cases, as only about one-third of resected specimens have adequate tumor-free margins. However, surgery still offers the only chance for cure if the lesions are resectable, and surgical (internal) drainage is also superior to external biliary drainage as a palliative procedure. Transplantation of the liver with the whole external hepatic biliary tree is advocated by some, provided there is no extrahepatic lymph node involvement.

Surgical resectability has advanced in several specialized centers to include partial hepatectomy and vascular reconstruction in the event of portal vein involvement. Extensive involvement of the vascular supply of the liver excludes surgical resection, although the patient may benefit from a biliary-drainage procedure. Exposure of a distended bile duct near the round ligament by limited dissection of the parenchyma of segment 3 enables a jejunal loop to be anastomosed to this area (segment 3 bypass).

1 | *Removal of Tumorous Bile Duct*

This diagram depicts a typical nodular or scirrhous-type Klatskin tumor involving the junction of the bile ducts, with possible invasion of the hepatic artery. Proximal to the tumor, the bile ducts are distended and easily identifiable, particularly if preoperative stenting has been performed (see page 178).

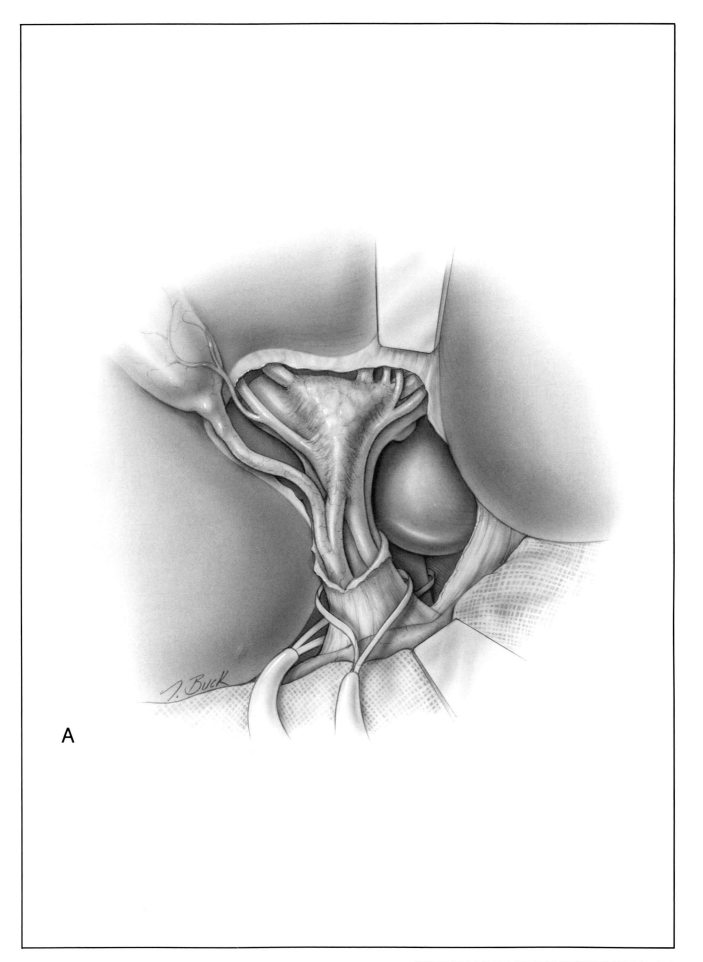

A

B

C

Endoscopic assessment with endoscopic retrograde cholangiopancreatography (ERCP) is invaluable. It gives access to histologic confirmation of the tumor and allows for the placement of biliary stents into both ducts. Optimal conditions are achieved when bilateral stenting is accomplished. Pigtail catheters facilitate bilateral decompression and drainage of the biliary tree for several weeks. Relief of jaundice allows for a more radical surgical approach and reduces the incidence of infections from cholestasis. Both stents serve as a guide into the intrahepatic segments of the left and right bile ducts. In addition, they allow an estimate of the proximal end of the tumor involvement if the strictures can be passed.

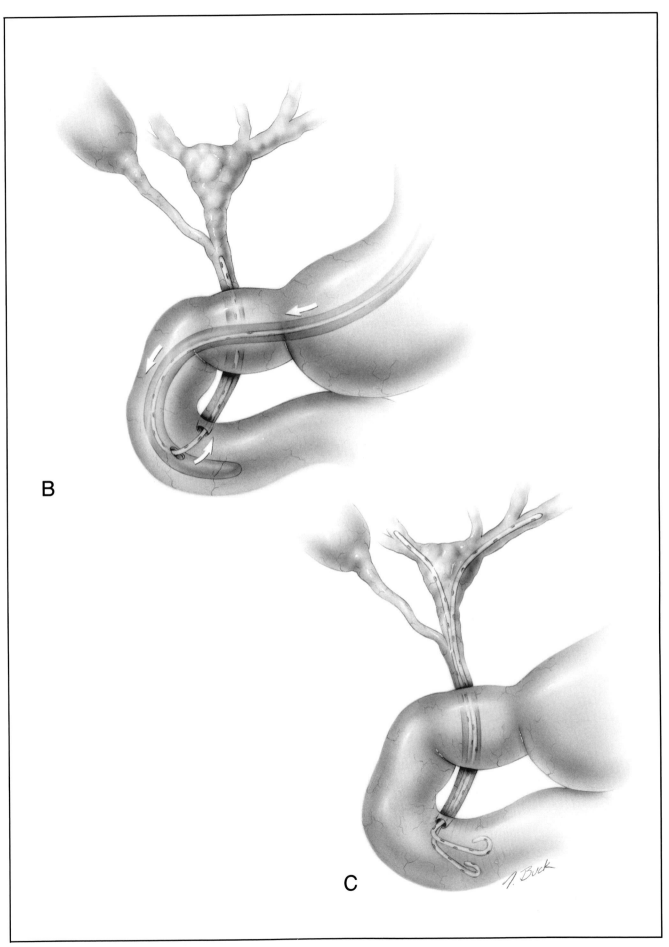

B

C

In some patients in whom endoscopic stenting is unsuccessful or unavailable, adequate biliary drainage can be accomplished via percutaneous placement of stents. Preoperative biliary drainage is highly recommended in these cases, and the Silastic stents should remain in place, as their positions serve to help the surgeon identify the bile ducts. Percutaneous cholangiography identifies the intrahepatic extend of the biliary lesion, thus, helping to assess operability preoperatively.

 If the Silastic stents are not draining, they should always be removed prior to surgical manipulation. The surgical incision is limited to a right subcostal approach until full assessment of the tumor and the possibility of resection has been made. The incision can always be extended if radical resection is indicated.

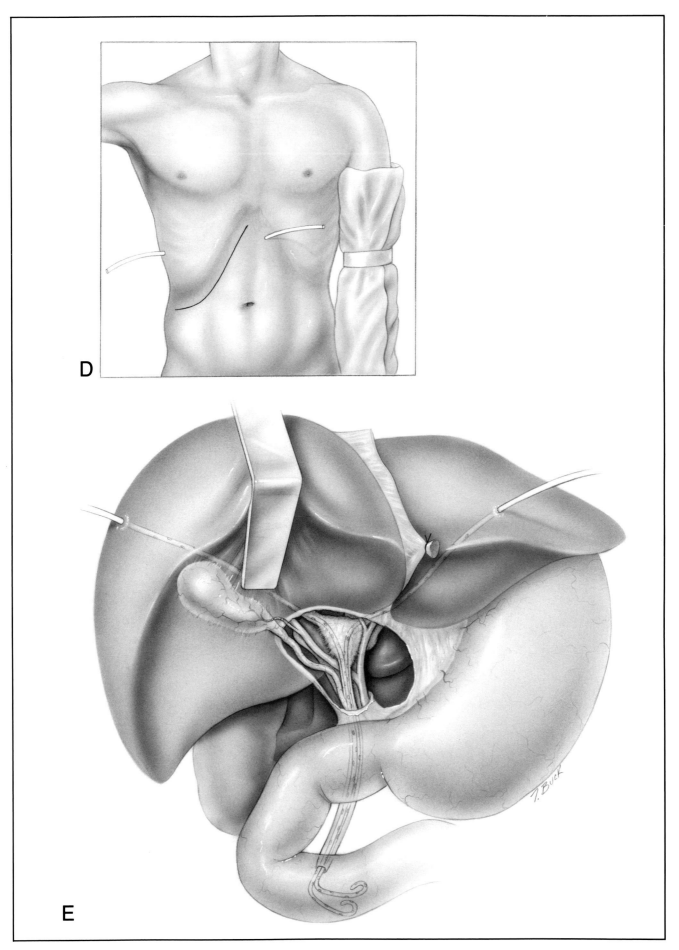

The dissection starts with exposure of the Calot's triangle; the hepatoduodenal ligament is fully palpated for tumor. Lymph nodes in this ligament are identified and sent for frozen section so the stage of the tumor can be assessed histologically, although only rarely are these lymph nodes involved. The tumor and, most importantly, the upper extent of the tumor should be palpated. If normal ducts can be felt above the tumor, then resectability is almost ensured. Once a decision has been made to proceed with the resection, tourniquets are placed around the hepatoduodenal ligament and the inferior vena cava for vascular control. The common bile duct is identified and divided close to the duodenum. Should a stent be in place, this is also cut and the distal end removed. The distal bile duct is carefully oversewn to avoid leakage of duodenal contents.

G Isolation of the common ducts starts with a routine cholecystectomy and identification of the right hepatic artery. The common duct is lifted toward the surface of the liver to allow preparation along the common hepatic artery. Usually the tumor does not penetrate the artery, and a plane can be dissected between the tumor and the adventitia. However, if both arteries are involved in the tumor and no plane is definable, we consider the situation to be unresectable. Occasionally, one artery can be preserved, and the possibility of performing a hepatectomy in association with excision of the tumor should be considered. The tumor is in close contact with the portal vein, but usually they can be separated relatively easily. Even if a small segment of the portal vein is involved in the hilar area, this can be resected with the tumor and the defect repaired with a venous/Gore-Tex patch. Resectability on the left side of the tumor is sometimes difficult to assess, because the artery runs on top of the bile duct. This area needs careful dissection, so that tumor clearance can be achieved.

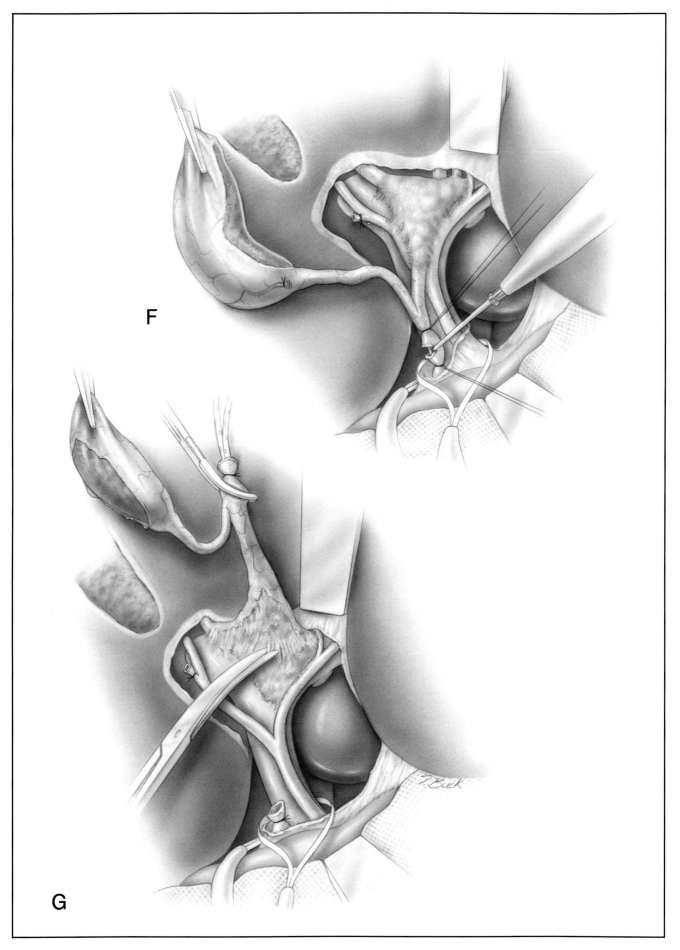

F

G

H Once the tumor is mobilized and the upper margins have been clearly defined, the formal dissection of the parenchyma can begin. Excision of the tumor starts with incision into the normal liver tissue of the quadrate lobe surrounding the tumor. Initial penetration of the parenchyma by electrocautery is required to fully excise the lesion. It is necessary to start on one side and clear the field of tumor tissue by dividing the vessels and even the bile ducts of the second and third order going to the hilum. Bleeding sites have to be suture-ligated until a reasonable cavity with a tumor-free margin of some millimeters has been created.

I The left hepatic ducts need to be followed close to the round ligament until the tumor can be approached posteriorly. Usually, the left median branch of the portal vein and the branch of the left hepatic artery need to be suture-ligated with 5-0 atraumatic monofilament suture. Within the large excavation, several orifices of small bile ducts open onto the surface. Frozen sections must be obtained from their margins to exclude residual tumor.

J A close-up view demonstrates how several bile ducts are sutured together to prepare a mucosa-mucosa anastomosis between the bile ducts and an isolated jejunal loop. Since most of the bile ducts are dilated due to the previous obstruction, the approximation of bile ducts becomes feasible. The cavity must be examined carefully to identify all the cut bile ducts.

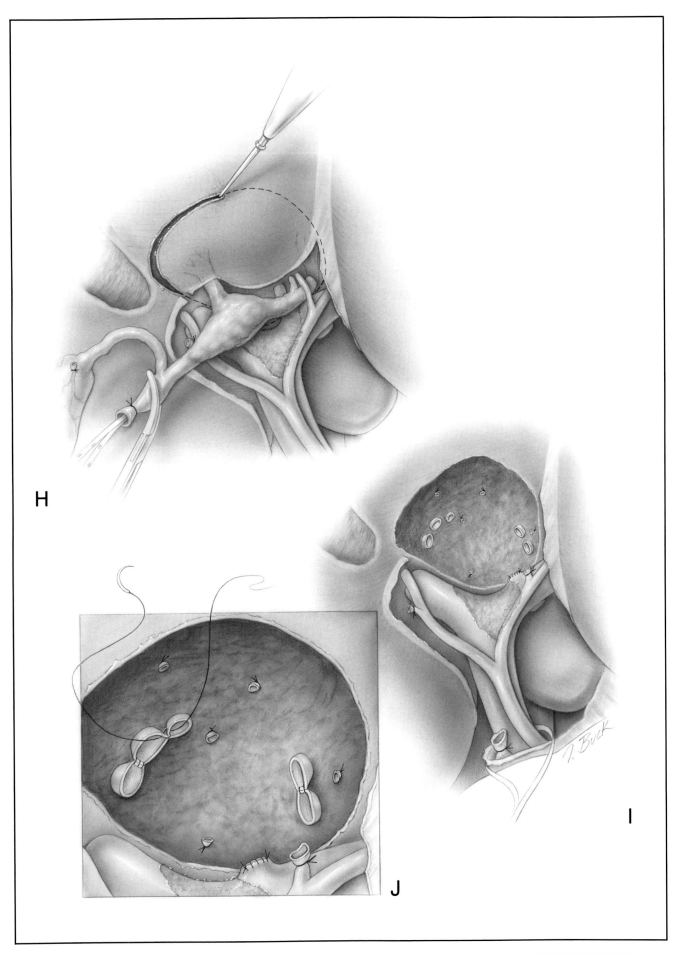

H

I

J

T. Buck

A Roux-en-Y loop is brought up and an end-to-side anastomosis prepared. The bile ducts are approximated as much as possible with interrupted sutures, usually the left ducts can form one group and the right ones another. Occasionally, a posterior bile duct draining the caudate lobe may have to be anastomosed to the loop separately. In this drawing, two separate confluences have been prepared, necessitating two enterotomies in the bowel loop. Following completion of the posterior line of interrupted sutures, the loop is brought up toward the hilum and the sutures tied. The anterior wall is then completed; the loop should lie snugly in the cavity. When a mucosa-mucosa anastomosis has been safely performed, providing there is no residual tumor, stenting of these anastomoses is not mandatory, and probably not necessary.

The hepaticojejunostomies are completed with a Roux-en-Y loop of at least 40 cm in length. Extreme care must be taken to avoid any leakage from this cavity from small ducts which may have been overlooked. This area is drained thoroughly.

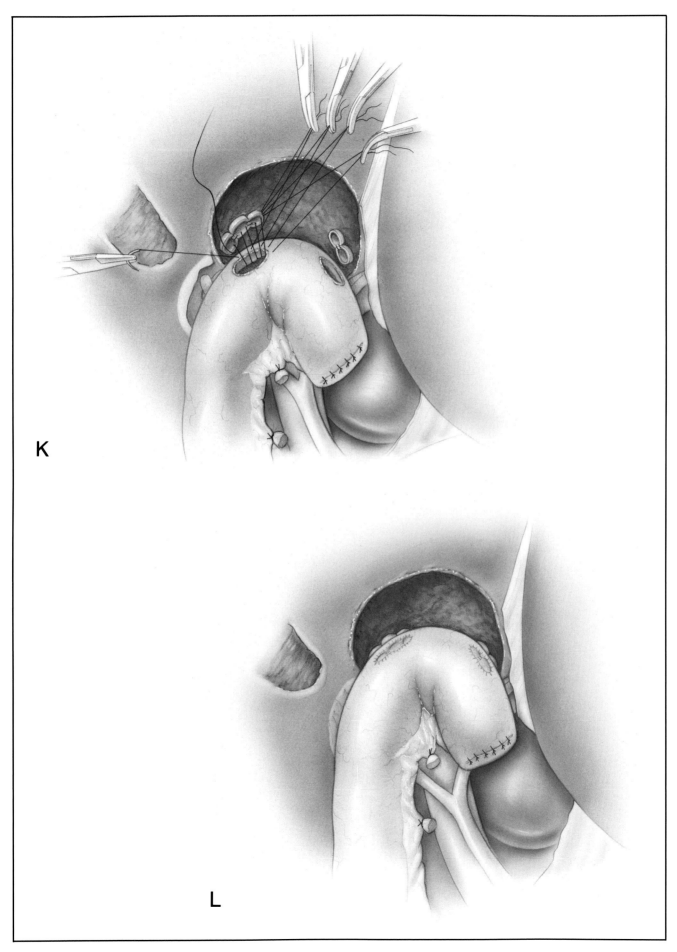

K

L

In cases of incomplete resection, when tumor remains at the margin of resection or along the portal vein and the caudate lobe, bilateral internal stenting is required in order to prevent recurrent obstruction in the near future. A special flexible spear is used for intubation of both sides of the major bile ducts. The flexible spear is advanced into a major bile duct and pushed through the parenchyma of the liver to come out through the liver capsule. Silastic tubes can then be attached to the end of the introducer, which is pulled through the liver until the tubes are exteriorized and the holes in the tubes lie across the anastomotic site. Often, a major duct to the right lobe as well as a major orifice into the left lobe require transparenchymal stenting.

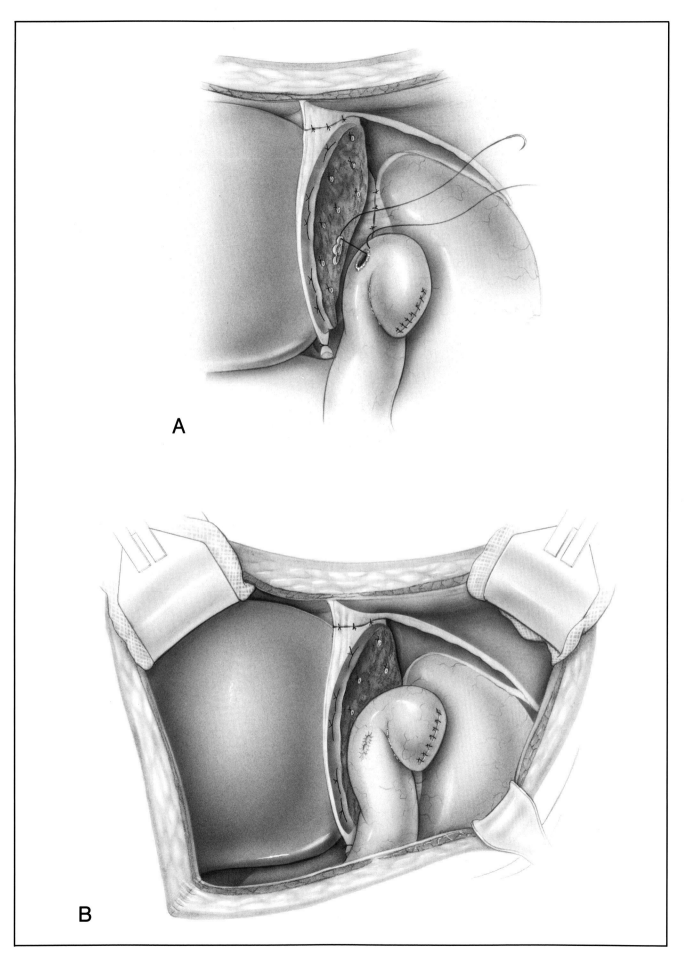

A

B

C

D

The median left segment has been removed, as described on page 96. The biliary elements from the right lobe and the left lateral segment are identified, but not suture-ligated. The Roux-en-Y loop is placed into the cavity and incisions made on the surface of the loop adjacent to the bile ducts. The posterior wall of one duct (or ductal system) is anastomosed first, followed by the corresponding anterior wall. The remaining ducts are sutured in turn, using interrupted 5-0 monofilament thread. The anastomoses and the cut surfaces of the liver are drained adequately.

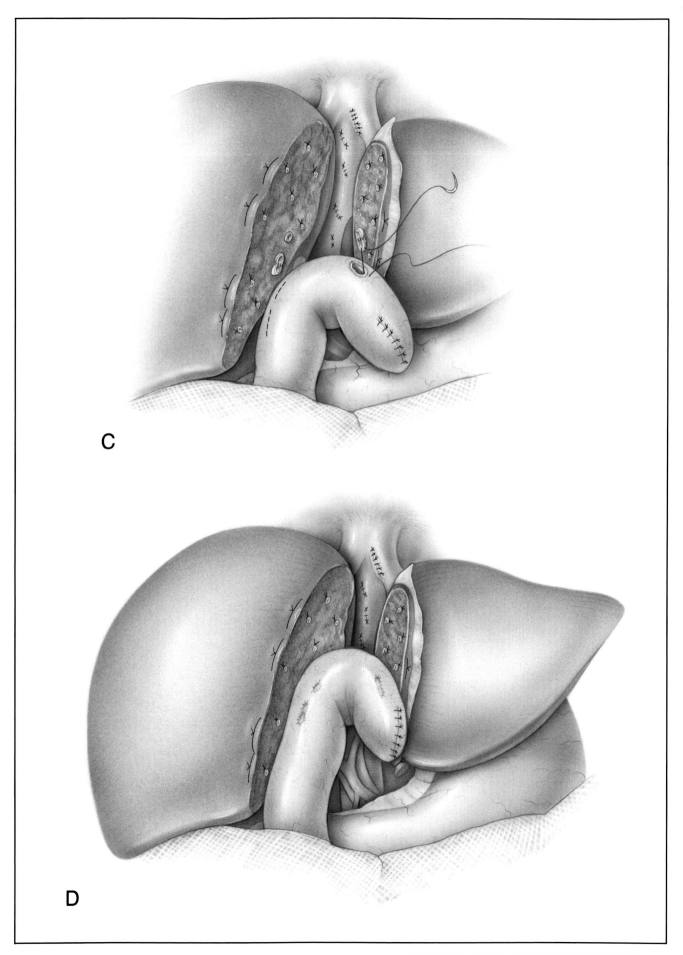

C

D

Trauma

There has been a revival of more conservative approaches in treating hepatic injuries over the past several years, and perihepatic packing has regained its popularity. Aggressive interventional surgery using atriocaval shunts is not generally beneficial, and certainly not applicable in the majority of cases, although its application is included in this chapter for completeness. Most liver injuries require little (if any) surgical treatment, and even the deepest injuries can require surprisingly little surgical intervention. Penetrating trauma is generally easier to manage than blunt trauma, which may be associated with deep stellate fractures within the liver. Procedures available to most competent surgeons are outlined in this chapter.

When a patient is suspected of having liver trauma, the abdomen is opened through a long midline incision that allows access to all visceral contents. Should there be a major liver laceration that requires surgical repair, the incision is extended laterally to the right, and even into the chest. If the abdomen is full of blood, it is quickly aspirated and all four quadrants of the abdomen packed firmly until cardiovascular stability is achieved, at which time the different packs can be removed carefully and the viscera examined systematically.

1 | *Capsular and Deep Stellate Wounds*

 Superficial capsular tears do not need definitive surgical treatment. The liver surface should be inspected and the lacerations very gently examined for their depth. No sutures are required, although temporary compression with abdominal packs may stop oozing. Application of hemostatic dressings may be beneficial, but electrocautery is very rarely indicated.

 Occasionally, large stellate fractures occur across the dome of the liver, but at the time of laparotomy there is little or no bleeding. If there is a blood clot in the depth of the fracture, it should not be disturbed. These fractures, once stabilized, should be covered with omentum, if available, and a soft plastic drain inserted into the cavity. Suturing the surfaces together is usually unsuccessful, and may cause additional bleeding.

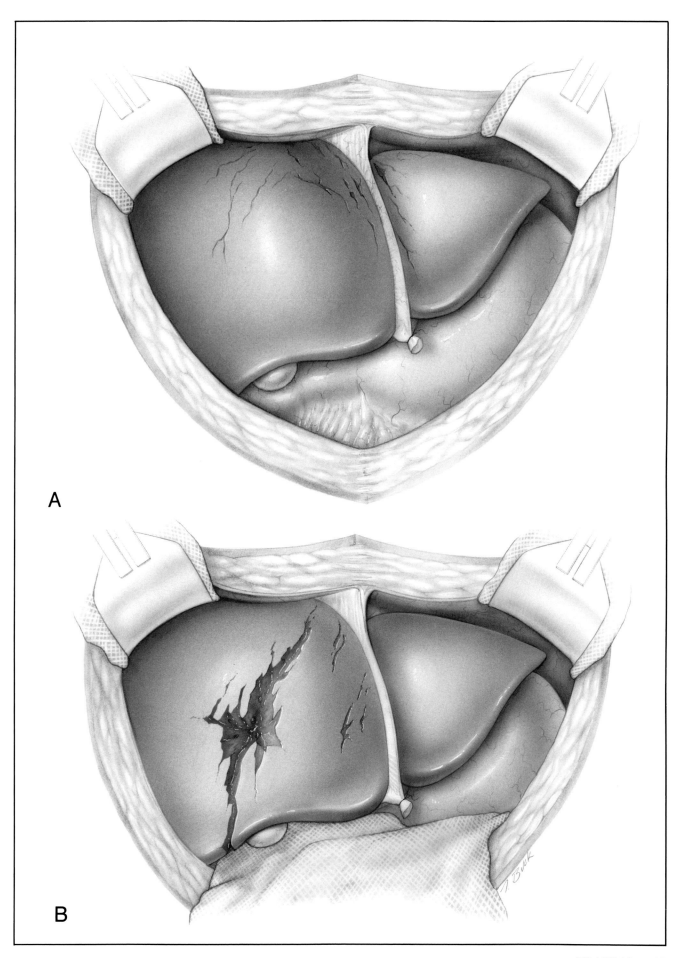

A

B

If there is continued bleeding from the fracture site, pressure should be applied to compress the liver, and the triangular ligaments should be divided. This helps to apply the compression in the appropriate fashion and gives access to the posterior surface, should bimanual compression be necessary to arrest hemorrhage.

 If the bleeding shows no sign of stopping, the fracture site must be explored. Remember: deep tears in the liver may affect major branches of the portal vein, which can bleed torrentially. A tourniquet around the hepatoduodenal ligament is mandatory before such exploration. Using gentle exploration with a straight arterial forceps, individual vessels and bile ducts can be suture-ligated under direct vision. For better access, part of the liver may have to be debrided in a nonanatomic resection.

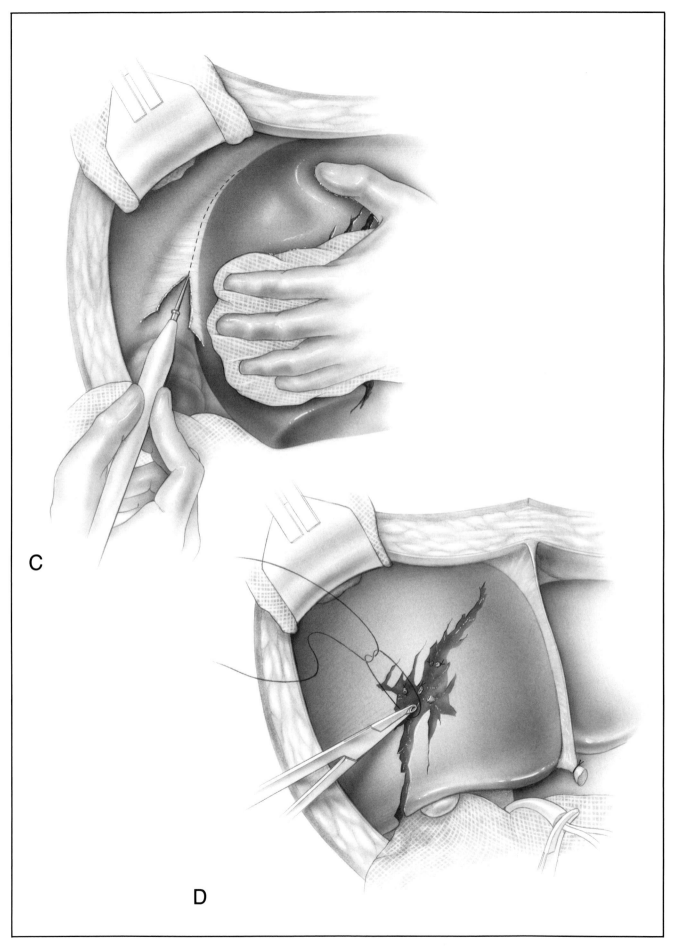

C

D

Once the bleeding is controlled or improved, the site is left alone and soft Silastic drains placed into the cavity. Omentum should be mobilized and secured into the fracture also. If the bleeding has been difficult to control, or there is continued oozing from deep within the rent, then packing is advocated. The abdominal packs must be placed extremely carefully and with great forethought. After full mobilization of the liver, the packs are placed sequentially from beneath the liver to its anterior surface. To provide even compression, the packs must be placed flat and not simply shoved unevenly into the subdiaphragmatic space. The packs are left in place for 48 hours and gently removed at relaparotomy.

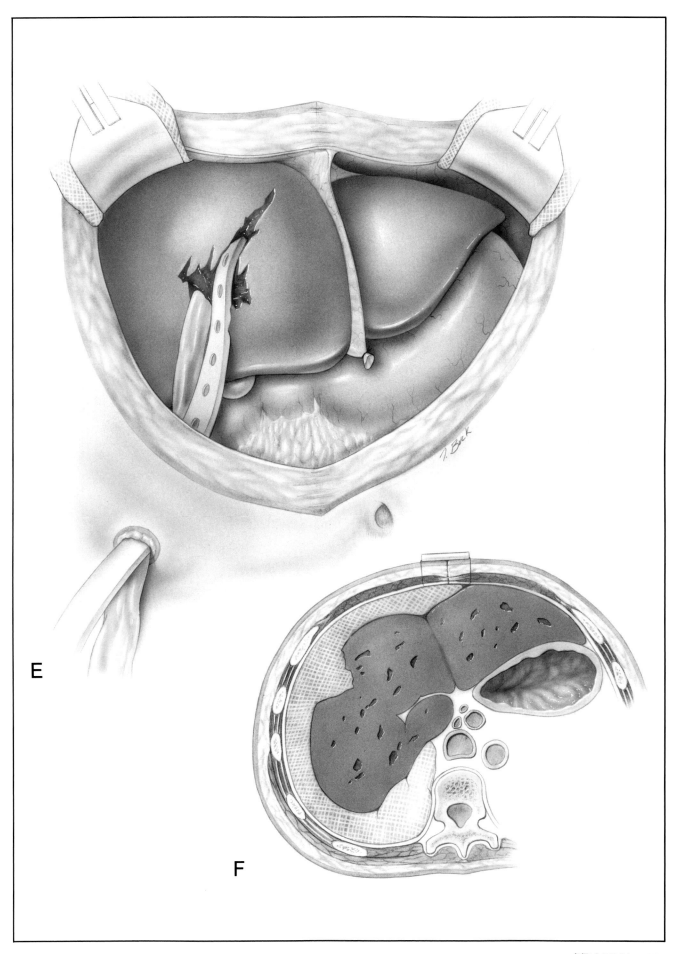

E

F

2 | *Stellate Wound Over Dome of Liver Including Trauma to Hepatic Vein*

A   Deep tears in the liver may involve one or more of the retrohepatic veins or the hepatic vein–cava complex. We would advocate that, if careful packing can control the bleeding, this area should not be explored and the packs can be removed at 48 hours. Even the most sizable tears in these veins can be controlled with diligent perihepatic packing.

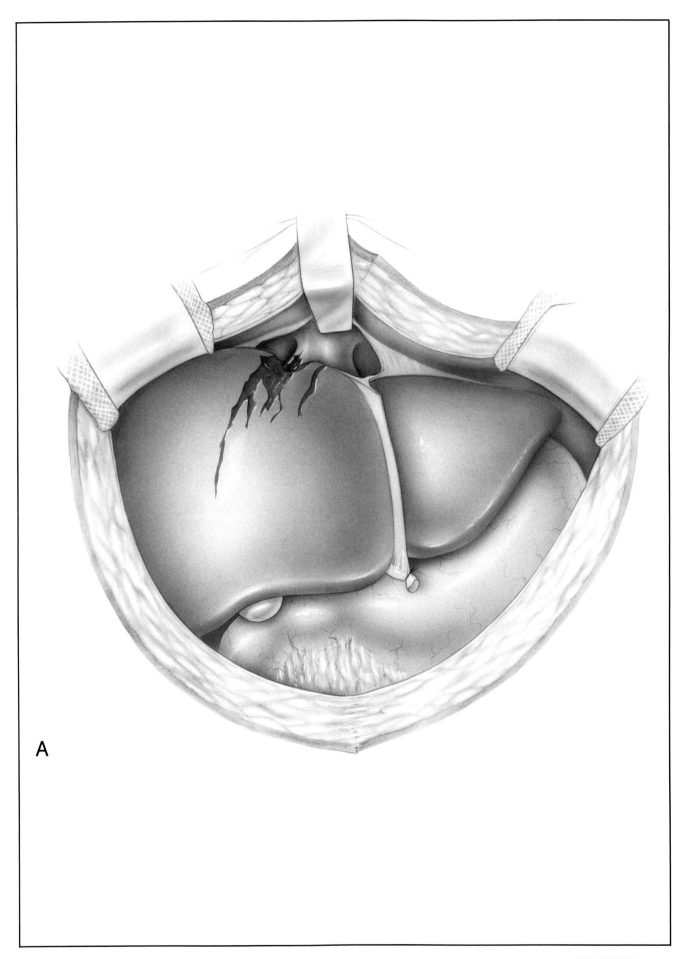

A

B In rare circumstances, the hemorrhaging is not controlled with compression and packing, and attempts at suturing are unrewarding. A final option available to the experienced liver surgeon should major bleeding persist is shown here. It demonstrates the insertion of an atriocaval shunt. While one assistant uses bimanual compression to the liver, both the infrahepatic cava and the hepatoduodenal ligament are slinged and occluded with tourniquets. The chest is opened through a median sternotomy and the pericardium incised. A pursestring suture is placed in the right atrial appendage and a large Silastic tube is passed through the heart to below the renal veins. Side holes in the tube allow blood to return to the right atrium from the cava. Extra tourniquets are placed around the intrathoracic inferior cava to secure hemostasis. Apart from a small number of lumbar veins, the liver is completely isolated and hemorrhage should cease. The liver parenchyma can be explored and the deep veins either repaired or suture-ligated. This procedure is associated with a 90 percent mortality, and is only done in desperate situations.

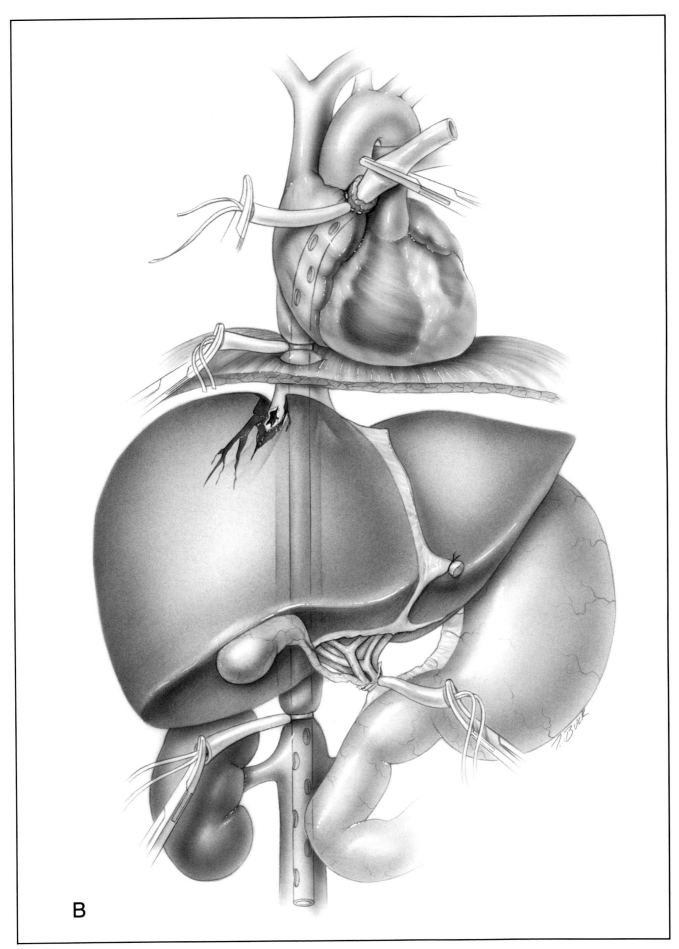

B

C

Once the lacerations have been controlled, the area should be carefully packed to produce uniform compression around the liver. The tourniquets are released very slowly to ensure hemorrhage is controlled. The tube is removed, and the cardiotomy closed.

In rare instances following frustrated attempts to control bleeding, although circulation can still be maintained, a complete excision of the lacerated organ can be performed resulting in an hepatic patient. The inferior vena cava has to be bridged by an interposition graft and a portacaval end-to-side shunt has to be constructed. Thus, within a period of 36 hours, a liver transplant needs to be performed.

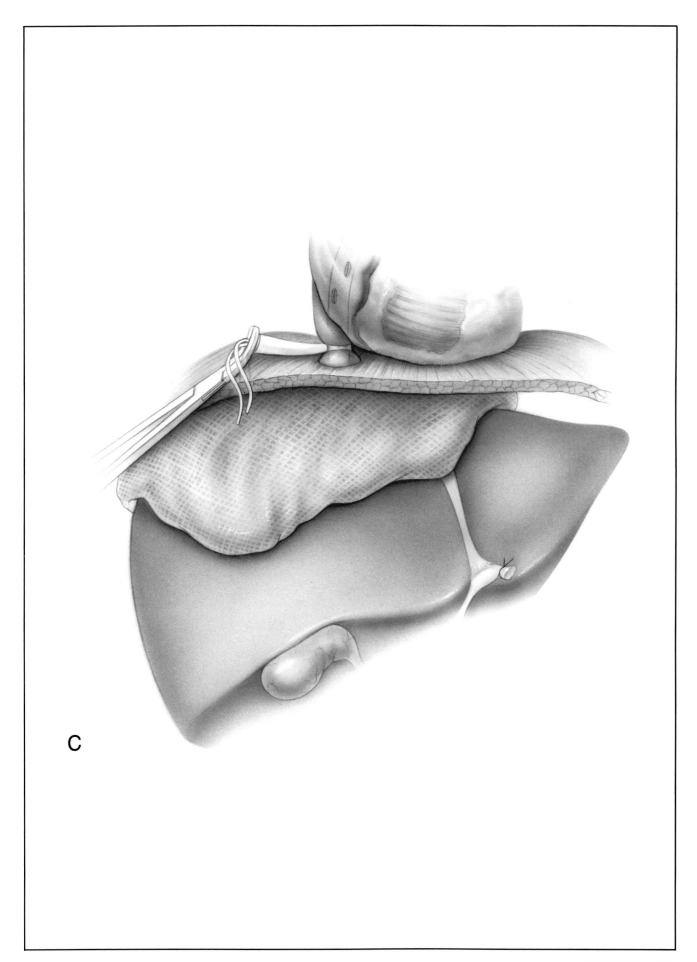

C

Drainage of Abscesses and Cysts

1 | *Abscesses*

In the Western world, hepatic abscesses are usually secondary to intra-abdominal sepsis, and occur either following intestinal surgery or as a consequence of cholecystitis/cholangitis, appendicitis, or chronic inflammatory disorders of the bowel. Occasionally they can be secondary to septicemic episodes, although they can occur spontaneously without any apparent cause and can be multifocal, multilocular, or solitary. Worldwide, the most common cause is amoebic infection. Abscesses should also be suspected in any patient who has persistent fever of unknown origin, and who is diagnosed by liver ultrasound and computed tomography (CT).

A

B

A subcostal incision will be adequate for the majority of cases; if the abscesses are located in the right lobe, this incision should be extended to the midaxillary line. If there is any doubt regarding the exact location of the collection, then intraoperative ultrasound is mandatory.

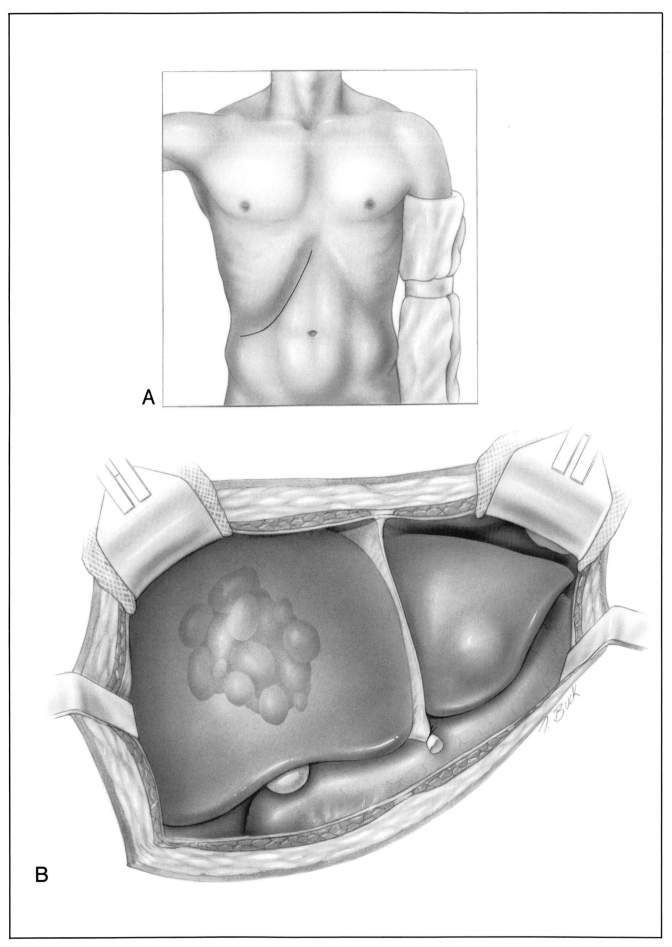

C
D
E
F

The liver should be mobilized sufficiently to enable packs to be placed around the operative field. If the abscesses are multifocal and there is risk of spillage, the packs should be soaked in Betadine prior to placement. Initially, an anaerobic culture can be obtained through needle aspiration, using a large syringe and a large needle. Preferably, the whole abscess cavity should be emptied in this manner. Once emptied, the abscess wall is incised with electrocautery and further culture swabs are taken. The contents of the cavity must be fully aspirated and the loculations broken down with the index finger. No attempt should be made to perform a pericystectomy in these patients, as it is impossible and can cause lethal hemorrhage. The roof of the abscess must be fully excised and sent for histologic examination. The cavity should be washed with Betadine and a soft Silastic drain inserted and secured before wound closure.

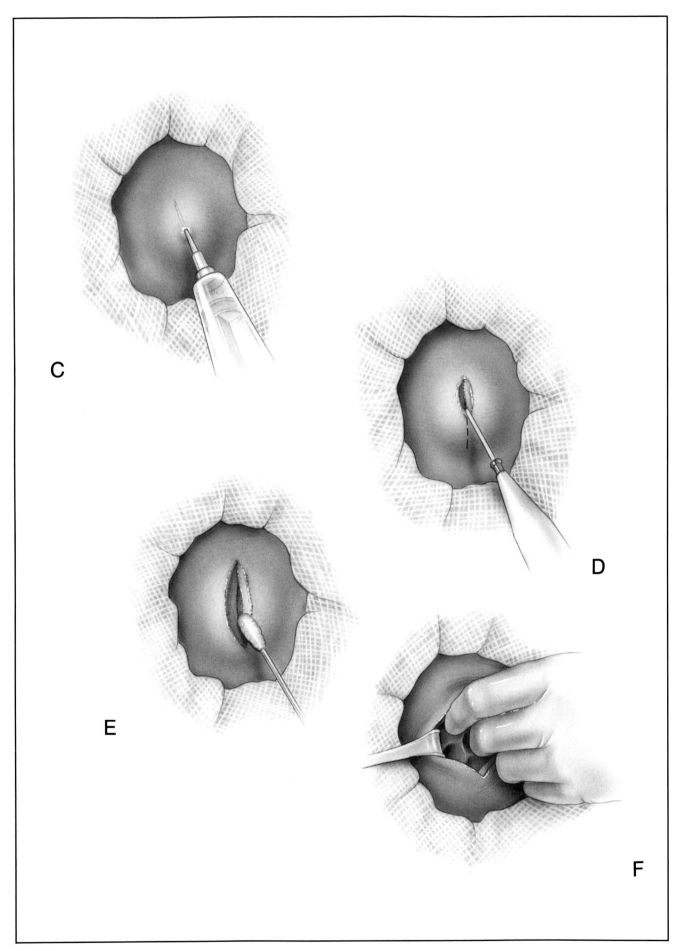

G
H
I

Multilocular abscess cavities are approached in the same way. Needle aspiration is attempted, and as much of the contents as possible emptied before surgical exploration. Wide deroofing is advised, and all loculations must be broken down. The contents of the cavity must be removed and the cavity flushed with Betadine and saline solution.

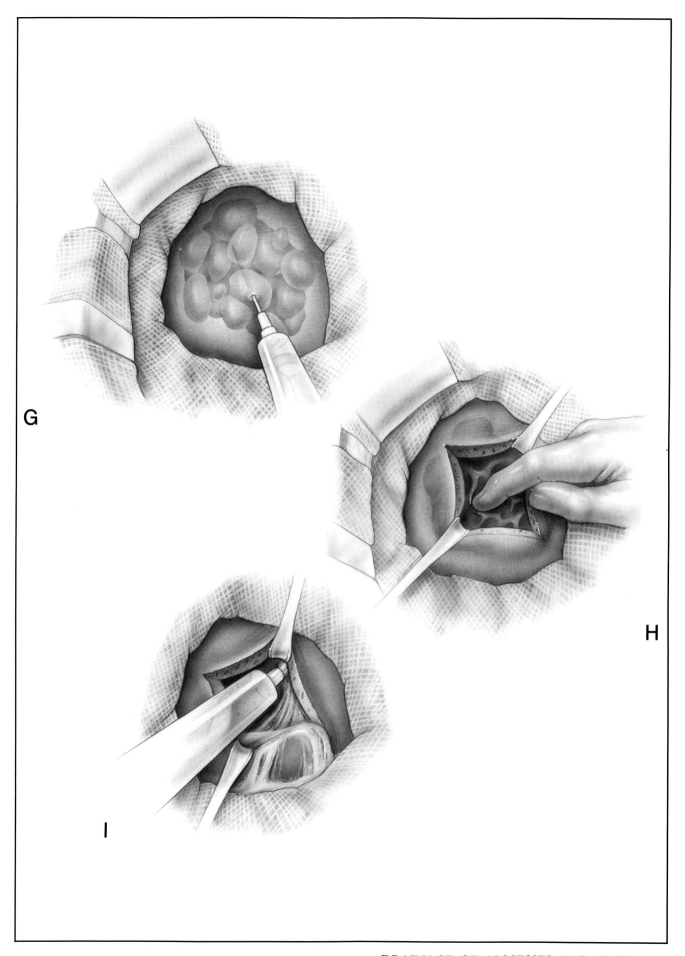

G

H

I

J As long as the cavity is completely de-roofed and adequately drained, most abscesses will heal. Soft drains must be inserted into the cavity and secured. Hemostasis from the cut margin of the liver is secured with electrocautery, although mattress sutures may be necessary if the cavity wall is very thick.

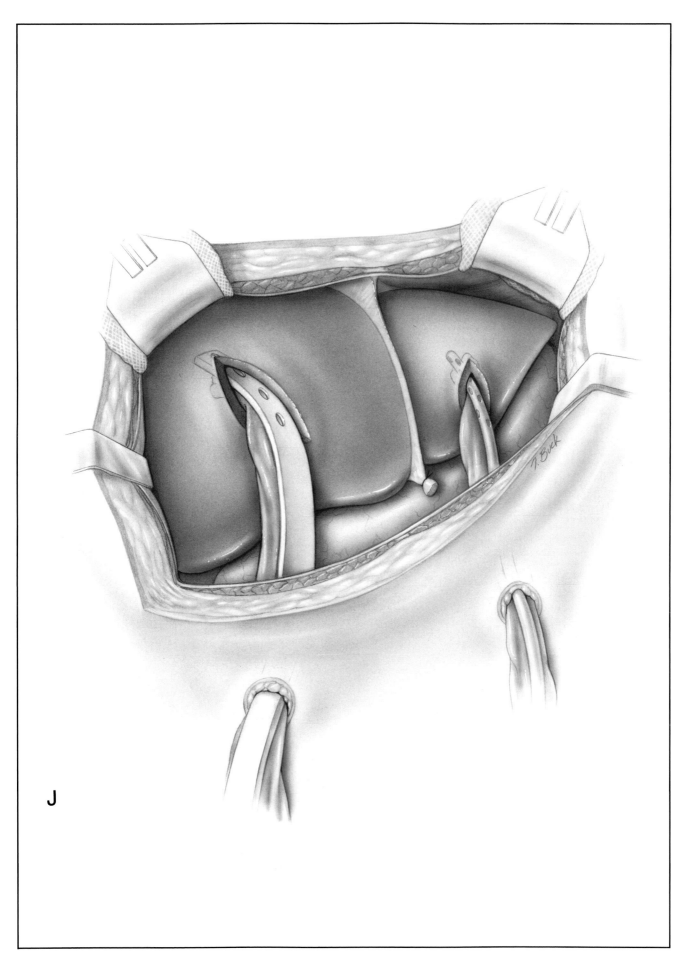

J

Alternatively, particularly when the cavity is thin-walled and contains little or no debris, parts of the greater omentum can be mobilized and sutured in place. Care must be taken that the omental flaps are not under tension. Drains are still advised, and can be inserted into the cavity between the sutures.

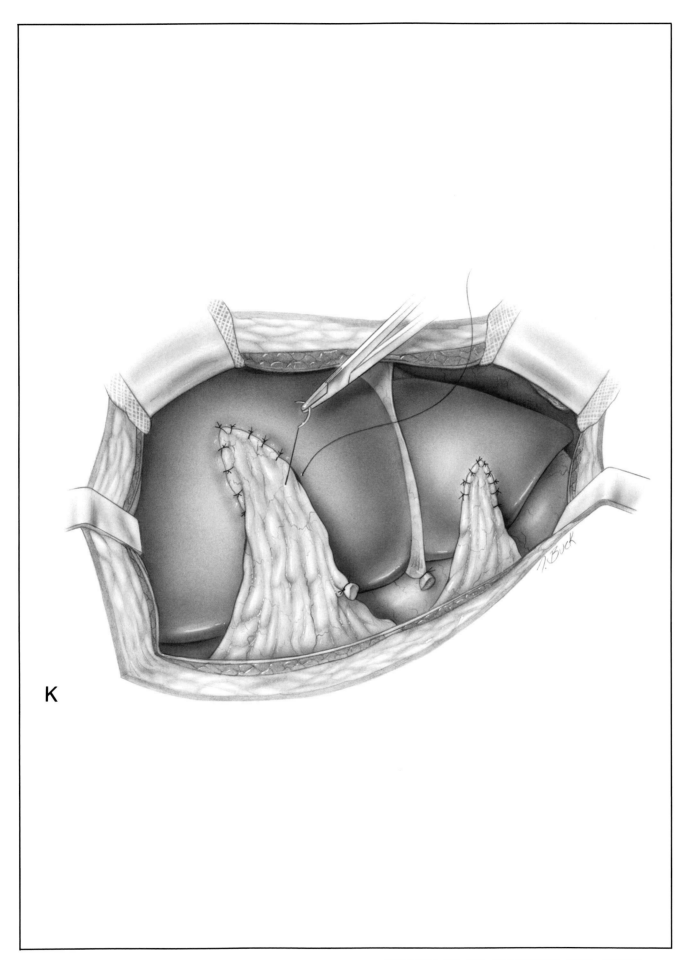

K

2 | *Cysts*

Polycystic liver disease is a rare condition, and can present patients with several problems. Generally, their symptoms are mild, with complaints of a fullness or dragging sensation in the abdomen. If the cysts are multiple and occupy most of the liver, patients can gradually develop liver failure and require transplantation. Simple solitary cysts should be deroofed using laparoscopic techniques, but patients with polycystic livers often have adhesions from their liver to the abdominal wall, making laparoscopic intervention difficult. Generally, the cysts should be deroofed at laparotomy. More recently, solitary cysts have been deroofed by laparoscopic surgical approach.

A
B

By the time the patient finally has surgery in an attempt to relieve the symptoms of polycystic liver disease, most of the liver is affected with cystic changes. The liver is mobilized carefully and the adhesions to the anterior abdominal wall are gently divided. Hemorrhage into the cysts is common and can make surgery difficult, not only because of scarring and fibrosis, but also because of continual bleeding from within the cysts.

Generally, as many of the cysts as possible should be incised and drained. This is done using electrocautery, although persistent bleeding sites may have to be underrun with mattress sutures. The liver in these patients may be friable and, because of impaired liver function, there may be associated coagulopathy. Hemostasis must be meticulous. Drains should always be inserted around the liver, because the large surface area exposed by multiple incisions may produce significant fluid and lymph.

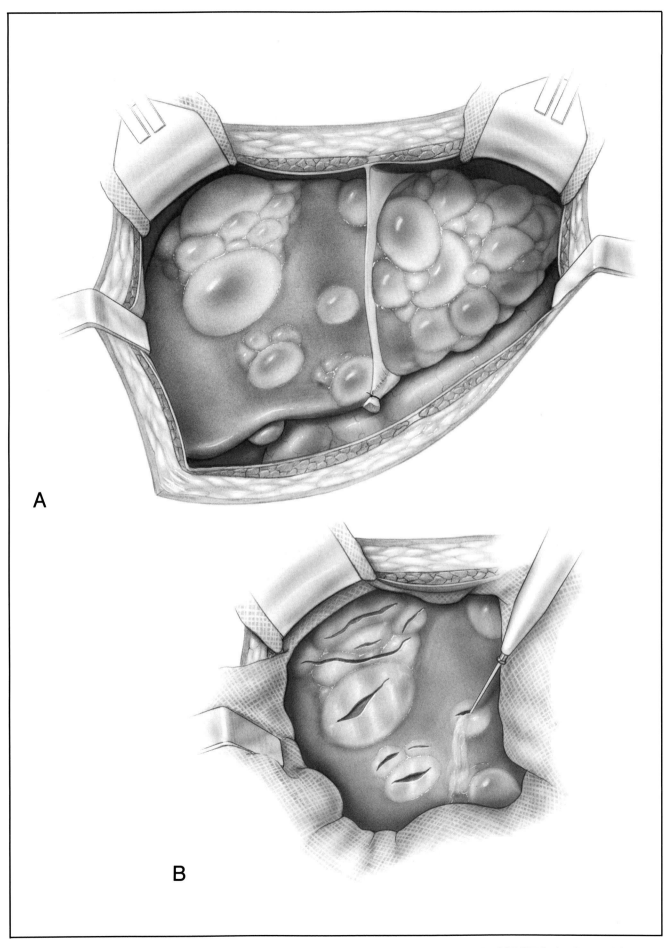

If there is a large cyst or a collection of cysts in the left lobe, and there is no demonstrable, viable liver tissue remaining, then a left lateral hepatectomy may be beneficial in reducing symptoms and preventing recurrence in that area. The techniques for resection are similar to that described in Chapter 1, although lateral hepatectomies in these particular patients can be quite demanding and should only be undertaken by an experienced hepatic surgeon. Again, hemostasis must be meticulous because of coagulopathy, and large drains need to be left in situ for several days.

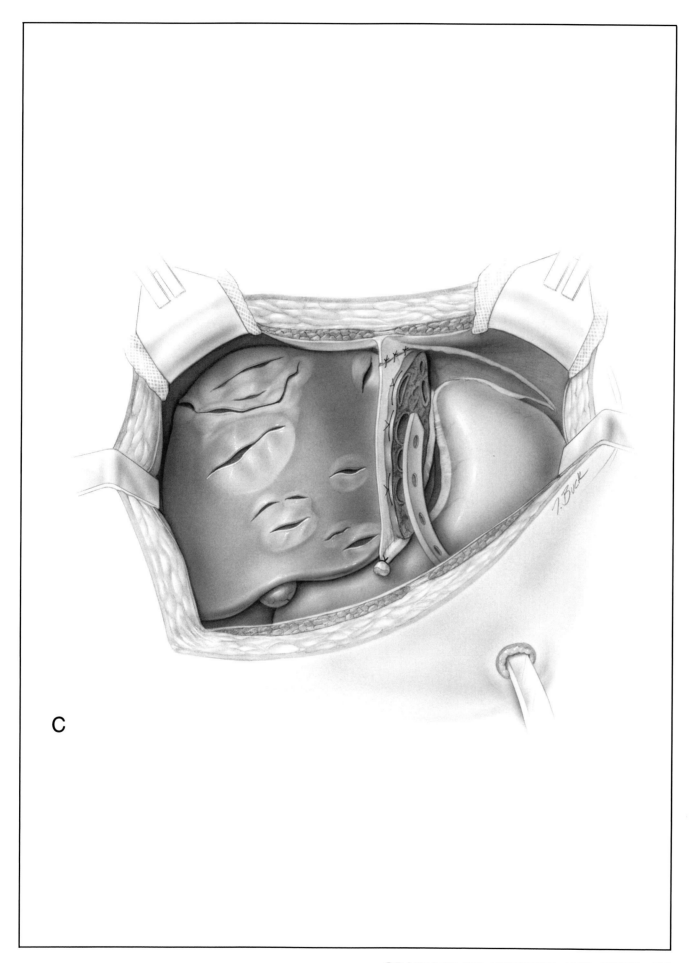

C

Index

Page numbers followed by f *represent figures.*

U

V